The New Atkins Diet Cookbook

100 Delicious And Easy-to-follow Low-Carb Recipes for Weight Loss And Wellness

Emily M. Wilson

Copyright © 2023 Emily M. Wilson

All rights reserved.

CONTENTS

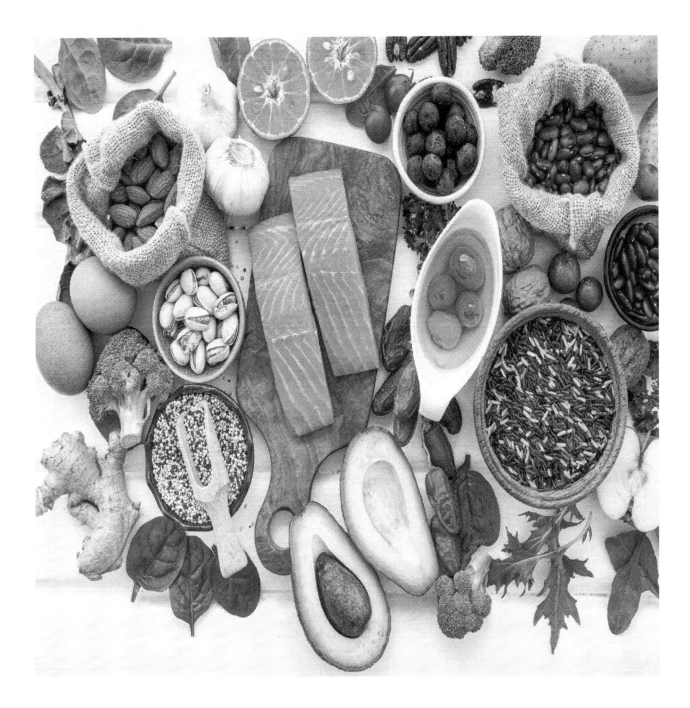

INTRODUCTION

In a world where fad diets come and go like passing trends, there emerges a beacon of science-backed nutrition that has stood the test of time - the Atkins Diet. Picture this: a path that leads you away from the labyrinth of calorie counting and deprivation, and instead, invites you to savor delicious, satisfying meals while achieving your health and weight goals.

Imagine waking up each morning with renewed vitality, mental clarity, and a body that exudes confidence. This isn't a fantasy; it's the promise that the Atkins Diet holds. It's a journey that empowers you to take control of your eating habits, transforming not only the number on the scale but also your overall well-being.

The Atkins Diet isn't just another fleeting dietary craze; it's a revolutionary approach that redefines the way we perceive nutrition and weight management. It's about embracing the foods that nature has gifted us - vibrant vegetables, lean proteins, and wholesome fats - while strategically moderating carbohydrate intake to unlock your body's incredible potential.

But what sets the Atkins Diet apart from the sea of diets clamoring for attention? Science. Solid, evidence-based science that dives deep into the metabolic processes within us. It's about understanding how our bodies react to different foods and tailoring our diet to work in harmony with our physiology.

The journey begins by embracing the concept of ketosis, where your body shifts from being a carbohydrate-burning machine to a fat-burning furnace. It's not about depriving yourself; it's about training your body to tap into its own energy reserves, shedding excess weight naturally and efficiently. And as the pounds melt away, something even more remarkable happens - your energy levels soar, your sugar cravings diminish, and your focus becomes laser-sharp.

But the Atkins Diet is not just a solo endeavor; it's a lifestyle that you can share with your loved ones. Imagine sitting around the table, savoring a delectable spread of nutrient-rich dishes, and knowing that you're not just enjoying a meal, but nourishing your body and soul.

In the chapters that follow, we'll delve into the science behind the Atkins Diet, guiding you through each phase of the journey. From the initial Induction phase that jumpstarts your metabolism, to the Balancing phase that refines your carb intake, and all the way to the Maintenance phase where you solidify your newfound vitality.

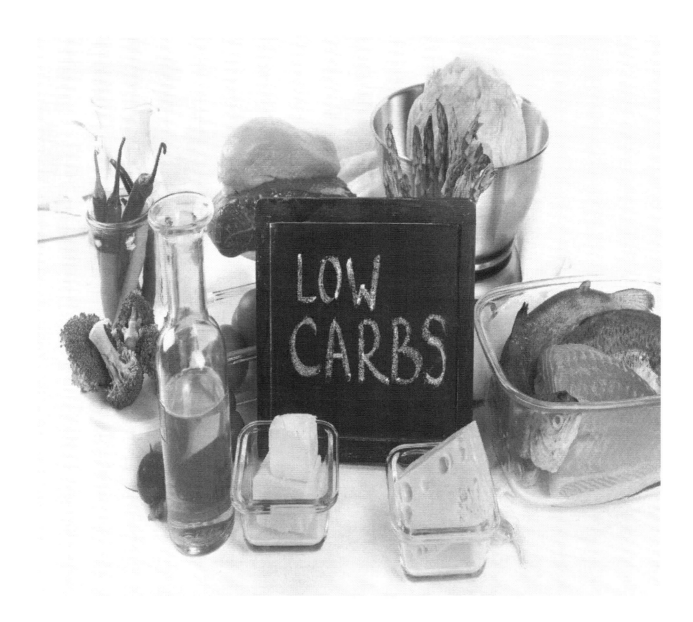

CHAPTER ONE: THE SCIENCE BEHIND THE ATKINS DIET

The Atkins Diet isn't just a dietary trend; it's grounded in the intricate science of how our bodies metabolize food. At its core lies the concept of ketosis - a metabolic state in which your body shifts from primarily burning carbohydrates for energy to utilizing stored fats. Understanding this science is pivotal to comprehending the transformative power of the Atkins Diet.

When carbohydrates are consumed, they break down into glucose, which your body converts into energy. Excess glucose is stored as fat. In a typical high-carb diet, your body relies heavily on glucose for energy, leaving little opportunity to tap into its fat stores.

The Atkins Diet disrupts this cycle by limiting carb intake, prompting the body to seek alternative energy sources. As carbs become scarcer, your liver begins converting fats into molecules called ketones, which serve as an efficient energy source. This metabolic shift not only triggers weight loss but also offers a range of health benefits.

Reducing carb intake and entering ketosis can stabilize blood sugar levels, an essential factor for diabetes management and prevention. It also curbs insulin production, reducing the risk of insulin resistance and related health issues. Furthermore, ketones are known to have a positive impact on brain function, potentially improving focus and mental clarity.

Getting Started with the Atkins Diet

Embarking on the Atkins Diet requires a well-informed, strategic approach. Before diving in, it's advisable to consult a healthcare professional to ensure the diet aligns with your health goals and medical history.

The diet operates in four distinct phases: Induction, Balancing, Pre-Maintenance, and Maintenance for Life. Each phase serves a specific purpose, guiding you toward your desired weight and health outcomes.

Induction Phase: The journey commences with the Induction phase. During this two-week period, carbohydrate intake is restricted to around 20-25 grams per day. This drastic reduction in carbs initiates ketosis, as your body adjusts to burning fat for fuel. Foods rich in healthy fats and proteins, such as meat, fish, eggs, and non-starchy vegetables, take center stage. This phase kickstarts weight loss, suppresses cravings, and regulates blood sugar levels.

Balancing Phase: Moving into the Balancing phase, you gradually introduce more carbohydrates, aiming to discover your personal carb tolerance while continuing to lose weight. This phase might last several weeks, depending on your progress and goals. It's about finding the sweet spot where weight loss is steady but sustainable. Nutrient-dense foods like berries, nuts, and certain grains make their way into your diet.

Pre-Maintenance Phase: The Pre-Maintenance phase is the bridge between active weight loss and lifelong maintenance. Here, you fine-tune your eating habits, experimenting with various carb levels until you're close to your goal weight. The focus is on identifying the carb intake that allows you to maintain your desired weight without feeling deprived.

Maintenance for Life: The ultimate destination is the Maintenance for Life phase, where you've achieved your target weight and embraced a sustainable eating pattern. Carbohydrates are no longer the enemy; rather, you've learned to choose healthier, whole-food options. The principles you've adopted become a part of your lifestyle, ensuring that your success endures.

To make your Atkins journey a triumph, here are a few key tips:

- Plan Meals: Create a meal plan that incorporates adequate protein, healthy fats, and low-carb vegetables. This balance keeps you satisfied and nourished.
- Stay Hydrated: Water is your ally. Hydration aids digestion and curbs cravings.

- Monitor Progress: Track your carb intake, weight loss, and how you feel. Adjust your approach accordingly.

- Incorporate Physical Activity: Exercise complements the diet, enhancing weight loss and overall health.

- Consult Professionals: Regular check-ins with healthcare and nutritional experts provide guidance and ensure you're on the right track.

Foods To Eat And Avoid On The Atkins Diet

The Atkins Diet is centered around strategic food choices to promote weight loss and overall well-being. Here's a brief guide on foods to eat and foods to avoid:

Foods to Eat:

- **Proteins:** Include lean meats (chicken, turkey, and beef), fish, seafood, eggs, and tofu. These are essential for muscle health and satiety.

- **Healthy Fats:** Opt for sources like avocados, nuts, seeds, olive oil, and coconut oil. These fats support energy and brain function.

- **Non-Starchy Vegetables:** Load up on nutrient-rich options like leafy greens, broccoli, cauliflower, zucchini, peppers, and asparagus.

- **Berries:** Limited quantities of berries like strawberries, raspberries, and blueberries can satisfy your sweet tooth without spiking blood sugar.

- **Dairy:** Enjoy moderate portions of full-fat dairy products, such as Greek yogurt, cheese, and cream.

- **Nuts and Seeds:** Almonds, walnuts, chia seeds, and flaxseeds are great for snacking and adding crunch to your meals.

- **Low-Carb Sweeteners:** In moderation, use natural sweeteners like stevia, erythritol, and monk fruit to add sweetness without added carbs.

Foods to Avoid:

- **High-Sugar Foods:** Cut out sugary treats, candies, soda, and sugary snacks that can disrupt blood sugar levels.

- **Grains and Starchy Foods:** Avoid bread, pasta, rice, and other high-carb grains. Also, steer clear of starchy vegetables like potatoes.

- **Processed Foods:** Stay away from heavily processed foods, including packaged snacks, fast food, and pre-made meals.

- **Sugary Condiments:** Many condiments contain hidden sugars. Avoid ketchup, sweet dressings, and sauces high in added sugars.

- **High-Carb Fruits:** Limit high-carb fruits like bananas, grapes, and tropical fruits, as they can raise your carb intake.

- **Legumes:** Beans, lentils, and peas are relatively high in carbs and should be minimized.

- **Trans Fats:** Avoid foods with trans fats, often found in processed baked goods and margarine.

- **Alcohol:** Alcoholic beverages can hinder ketosis and add extra calories. If you choose to drink, do so in moderation.

Remember, the Atkins Diet emphasizes individualized carb intake based on the phase you're in. During the Induction phase, carbs are restricted, but they gradually increase as you progress. It's essential to read labels, track your intake, and focus on whole, nutrient-dense foods to make the most of this dietary approach.

CHAPTER TWO: RECIPES

BREAKFAST AND BRUNCH RECIPES

1. Avocado and Egg Breakfast Bowl

Servings: 1

Prep Time: 5 minutes

Cook Time: 10 minutes

Ingredients:

- 1 ripe avocado, halved and pitted
- 2 eggs
- Salt and pepper to taste
- Chopped fresh herbs (such as parsley or chives) for garnish

Instructions:

1. Preheat the oven to 375°F (190°C).
2. Scoop out a bit of flesh from each avocado half to create a larger well for the egg.
3. Place the avocado halves in a baking dish.
4. Crack an egg into each avocado half, taking care not to overflow.
5. Season with salt and pepper.
6. Bake for about 10 minutes or until the egg whites are set.
7. Garnish with chopped herbs and serve.

Nutritional Information:

Calories: 320 | Protein: 12g | Fat: 28g | Net Carbs: 4g | Fiber: 7g

Key Benefits: Avocado provides healthy fats and fiber, while eggs are a great source of protein.

Tips: Add some diced tomatoes or crumbled bacon on top for extra flavor.

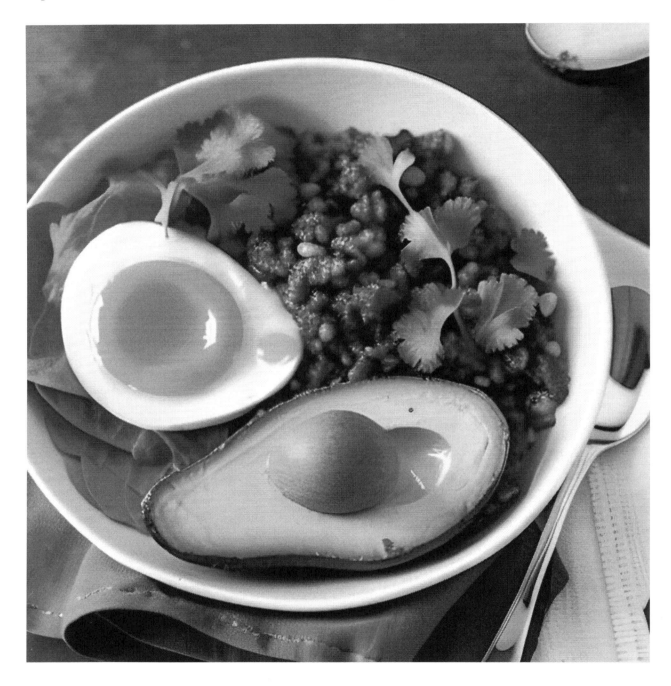

2. Spinach and Feta Omelette

Servings: 1

Prep Time: 5 minutes

Cook Time: 10 minutes

Ingredients:

- 3 eggs
- 1/2 cup fresh spinach, chopped
- 1/4 cup crumbled feta cheese
- Salt and pepper to taste
- 1 teaspoon olive oil

Instructions:

1. In a bowl, whisk the eggs with a pinch of salt and pepper.
2. Heat olive oil in a non-stick skillet over medium heat.
3. Add the chopped spinach and sauté until wilted.
4. Pour the whisked eggs into the skillet, swirling to cover the bottom.
5. Cook until the edges set, then sprinkle feta cheese over one half of the omelette.
6. Carefully fold the other half over the cheese.
7. Cook for another 2-3 minutes until the cheese melts and the omelette is cooked through.
8. Slide onto a plate and serve.

Nutritional Information:

Calories: 330 | Protein: 22g | Fat: 24g | Net Carbs: 3g | Fiber: 1g

Key Benefits: Spinach offers vitamins and minerals, while feta cheese contributes protein and flavor.

Tips: Add diced tomatoes or sautéed mushrooms for extra variety.

3. Coconut Flour Pancakes

Servings: 2-3

Prep Time: 10 minutes

Cook Time: 10 minutes

Ingredients:

- 1/4 cup coconut flour
- 4 eggs
- 1/4 cup unsweetened almond milk
- 1/2 teaspoon baking powder
- Pinch of salt
- Butter or coconut oil for cooking

Instructions:

1. In a bowl, whisk together eggs, almond milk, baking powder, and salt.
2. Gradually add the coconut flour while whisking to avoid lumps.
3. Heat a skillet over medium-low heat and add a small amount of butter or coconut oil.
4. Pour small amounts of batter onto the skillet to make pancakes.
5. Cook until bubbles form on the surface, then flip and cook the other side.
6. Repeat with the remaining batter.
7. Serve with your favorite toppings like sugar-free maple syrup and berries.

Nutritional Information:

Calories: 150 (per serving) | Protein: 8g | Fat: 10g | Net Carbs: 4g | Fiber: 3g

Key Benefits: Coconut flour is low in carbs and high in fiber, making it a great option for low-carb baking.

Tips: Customize with a dash of cinnamon or vanilla extract for added flavor.

4. Chia Seed Pudding

Servings: 2

Prep Time: 5 minutes (plus chilling time)

Ingredients:

- 1/4 cup chia seeds
- 1 cup unsweetened almond milk
- 1 teaspoon vanilla extract
- 1 tablespoon low-carb sweetener (stevia, erythritol, or monk fruit)
- Berries and chopped nuts for topping

Instructions:

1. In a bowl, mix chia seeds, almond milk, vanilla extract, and sweetener.
2. Stir well to prevent clumps, then let the mixture sit for 10 minutes.
3. Stir again to break up any clumps, then cover and refrigerate for at least 2 hours or overnight.
4. When ready to serve, divide the pudding into bowls and top with berries and chopped nuts.

Nutritional Information:

Calories: 180 (per serving) | Protein: 4g | Fat: 12g | Net Carbs: 7g | Fiber: 11g

Key Benefits: Chia seeds are rich in fiber and omega-3 fatty acids, providing a hearty and satisfying breakfast.

Tips: Experiment with different flavors by adding cocoa powder or a dash of cinnamon.

5. Bacon and Egg Breakfast Muffins

Servings: 4

Prep Time: 10 minutes

Cook Time: 20 minutes

Ingredients:

- 6 eggs
- 6 slices cooked bacon, crumbled
- 1/2 cup shredded cheddar cheese
- Salt and pepper to taste
- Chopped fresh chives for garnish

Instructions:

1. Preheat the oven to 350°F (175°C) and grease a muffin tin.
2. In a bowl, whisk eggs, crumbled bacon, shredded cheese, salt, and pepper.
3. Pour the mixture evenly into the muffin cups.
4. Bake for about 20 minutes or until the eggs are set and slightly golden.
5. Garnish with chopped chives and serve.

Nutritional Information:

Calories: 260 | Protein: 18g | Fat: 18g | Net Carbs: 1g | Fiber: 0g

Key Benefits: Eggs provide high-quality protein, while bacon adds flavor and healthy fats.

Tips: Add sautéed vegetables like bell peppers or spinach for added nutrients.

6. Greek Yogurt Parfait

Servings: 1

Prep Time: 5 minutes

Ingredients:

- 1/2 cup full-fat Greek yogurt
- 1/4 cup mixed berries (such as blueberries, raspberries, and strawberries)
- 2 tablespoons chopped nuts (almonds, walnuts, or pecans)

Instructions:

1. In a glass or bowl, layer Greek yogurt, mixed berries, and chopped nuts.
2. Repeat the layers.
3. Serve immediately.

Nutritional Information:

Calories: 250 | Protein: 12g | Fat: 17g | Net Carbs: 8g | Fiber: 4g

Key Benefits: Greek yogurt provides protein, probiotics, and calcium, while berries offer antioxidants and vitamins.

Tips: Use unsweetened yogurt and add a drizzle of natural sweetener like stevia if desired.

7. Zucchini and Cheese Fritters

Servings: 2-3

Prep Time: 15 minutes

Cook Time: 15 minutes

Ingredients:

- 2 medium zucchinis, grated and squeezed dry
- 1/2 cup grated Parmesan cheese
- 2 eggs
- 2 tablespoons coconut flour
- Salt and pepper to taste
- Olive oil for frying

Instructions:

1. In a bowl, combine grated zucchini, Parmesan cheese, eggs, coconut flour, salt, and pepper.
2. Heat olive oil in a skillet over medium heat.
3. Spoon small portions of the mixture onto the skillet and flatten with a spatula.
4. Cook for 3-4 minutes on each side or until golden brown.
5. Place the fritters on a paper towel to absorb excess oil.
6. Serve with a dollop of sour cream or Greek yogurt.

Nutritional Information:

Calories: 180 (per serving) | Protein: 12g | Fat: 11g | Net Carbs: 5g | Fiber: 2g

Key Benefits: Zucchini is low in carbs and high in vitamins, while cheese contributes protein and flavor.

Tips: Customize with herbs and spices like garlic powder or dried oregano.

8. Smoked Salmon and Cream Cheese Roll-Ups

Servings: 2

Prep Time: 10 minutes

Ingredients:

- 4 slices smoked salmon
- 4 tablespoons cream cheese
- 1 tablespoon capers
- Fresh dill for garnish

Instructions:

1. Lay out the smoked salmon slices on a clean surface.
2. Spread a tablespoon of cream cheese on each slice.
3. Sprinkle capers over the cream cheese.
4. Roll up the salmon slices and secure with toothpicks.
5. Garnish with fresh dill and serve.

Nutritional Information:

Calories: 200 (per serving) | Protein: 15g | Fat: 15g | Net Carbs: 2g | Fiber: 0g

Key Benefits: Smoked salmon provides omega-3 fatty acids and protein, while cream cheese adds creaminess.

Tips: Add slices of cucumber or avocado before rolling for extra freshness.

9. Cauliflower Hash Browns

Servings: 2-3

Prep Time: 15 minutes

Cook Time: 15 minutes

Ingredients:

- 2 cups grated cauliflower
- 1 egg
- 1/4 cup grated Parmesan cheese
- 1/4 teaspoon garlic powder
- Salt and pepper to taste
- Butter or olive oil for cooking

Instructions:

1. Place the grated cauliflower in a microwave-safe bowl and microwave for 2-3 minutes to soften.
2. Squeeze out excess moisture from the cauliflower using a clean kitchen towel.
3. In a bowl, mix the cauliflower, egg, Parmesan cheese, garlic powder, salt, and pepper.
4. Heat butter or olive oil in a skillet over medium heat.
5. Form the cauliflower mixture into patties and cook until golden brown on each side.
6. Serve with a dollop of sour cream or salsa.

Nutritional Information:

Calories: 120 (per serving) | Protein: 7g | Fat: 8g | Net Carbs: 3g | Fiber: 2g

Key Benefits: Cauliflower is a low-carb vegetable rich in vitamins and minerals, making it an excellent alternative to traditional hash browns.

Tips: Add grated cheddar cheese to the mixture for extra flavor and cheesiness.

10. Low-Carb Breakfast Burrito

Servings: 1

Prep Time: 10 minutes

Cook Time: 10 minutes

Ingredients:

- 2 large eggs
- 2 slices cooked bacon, chopped
- 1/4 cup diced bell peppers
- 1/4 cup diced onions
- 2 tablespoons shredded cheddar cheese
- Salt and pepper to taste
- Sliced avocado for topping

Instructions:

1. In a bowl, whisk the eggs with salt and pepper.
2. Heat a non-stick skillet over medium heat and add the diced peppers and onions.
3. Sauté until vegetables are tender, then add the chopped bacon.
4. Pour the whisked eggs into the skillet and scramble with the vegetables and bacon.
5. Once the eggs are cooked, sprinkle shredded cheddar cheese over the mixture.
6. Spoon the egg mixture onto a large lettuce leaf and roll it up like a burrito.
7. Top with sliced avocado and serve.

Nutritional Information:

Calories: 350 | Protein: 20g | Fat: 27g | Net Carbs: 4g | Fiber: 3g

Key Benefits: Bell peppers and onions provide vitamins and antioxidants, while avocado adds healthy fats.

Tips: Use a large cabbage leaf or collard green leaf as a sturdy wrap.

11. Almond Flour Waffles

Servings: 2-3

Prep Time: 10 minutes

Cook Time: 10 minutes

Ingredients:

- 1 cup almond flour
- 2 eggs
- 1/4 cup unsweetened almond milk
- 1/2 teaspoon baking powder
- Pinch of salt
- Butter or coconut oil for greasing

Instructions:

1. In a bowl, whisk together almond flour, eggs, almond milk, baking powder, and salt.
2. Preheat a waffle iron and grease it with butter or coconut oil.
3. Pour the batter onto the waffle iron and cook according to the manufacturer's instructions.
4. Repeat with the remaining batter.
5. Serve the waffles with sugar-free maple syrup and berries.

Nutritional Information:

Calories: 250 (per serving) | Protein: 10g | Fat: 20g | Net Carbs: 4g | Fiber: 2g

Key Benefits: Almond flour is low in carbs and high in healthy fats, providing a great alternative to traditional waffles.

Tips: Add a dash of cinnamon or vanilla extract to the batter for extra flavor.

12. Sausage and Veggie Breakfast Casserole

Servings: 4-6

Prep Time: 15 minutes

Cook Time: 40 minutes

Ingredients:

- 1/2 pound ground sausage, cooked and crumbled
- 1 cup diced bell peppers
- 1/2 cup diced onions
- 1 cup shredded cheddar cheese
- 6 eggs
- 1 cup heavy cream
- Salt and pepper to taste
- Chopped fresh parsley for garnish

Instructions:

1. Preheat the oven to 375°F (190°C) and grease a baking dish.
2. Spread the cooked sausage, diced peppers, and onions in the baking dish.
3. Sprinkle shredded cheddar cheese over the mixture.
4. In a bowl, whisk eggs, heavy cream, salt, and pepper.
5. Pour the egg mixture over the ingredients in the baking dish.
6. Bake for about 35-40 minutes or until the casserole is set and golden.
7. Garnish with chopped parsley before serving.

Nutritional Information:

Calories: 380 (per serving) | Protein: 18g | Fat: 31g | Net Carbs: 4g | Fiber: 1g

Key Benefits: Bell peppers and onions provide vitamins and antioxidants, while eggs and sausage offer protein and healthy fats.

Tips: Customize with your favorite vegetables like spinach or mushrooms.

13. Green Smoothie Bowl

Servings: 1

Prep Time: 5 minutes

Ingredients:

- 1 cup unsweetened almond milk
- 1 cup fresh spinach
- 1/2 avocado
- 1/4 cup frozen berries
- 1 scoop low-carb protein powder (optional)
- Toppings: chia seeds, sliced almonds, shredded coconut

Instructions:

1. In a blender, combine almond milk, spinach, avocado, frozen berries, and protein powder.
2. Blend until smooth and creamy.
3. Pour the smoothie into a bowl.
4. Top with chia seeds, sliced almonds, and shredded coconut.

Nutritional Information:

Calories: 300 | Protein: 15g | Fat: 22g | Net Carbs: 8g | Fiber: 10g

Key Benefits: Spinach provides vitamins and minerals, avocado adds healthy fats, and berries offer antioxidants.

Tips: Adjust the thickness by adding more or less almond milk.

14. Mushroom and Goat Cheese Frittata

Servings: 4-6

Prep Time: 15 minutes

Cook Time: 25 minutes

Ingredients:

- 8 eggs
- 1 cup sliced mushrooms
- 1/4 cup crumbled goat cheese
- 1/4 cup chopped fresh herbs (such as thyme or parsley)
- Salt and pepper to taste
- Olive oil for cooking

Instructions:

1. Preheat the oven to 375°F (190°C).
2. In a bowl, whisk eggs, salt, pepper, and chopped herbs.
3. Heat olive oil in an oven-safe skillet over medium heat.
4. Add sliced mushrooms and sauté until tender.
5. Pour the whisked eggs into the skillet, distributing mushrooms evenly.
6. Crumble goat cheese over the eggs.
7. Cook on the stovetop for a few minutes until the edges set.
8. Transfer the skillet to the preheated oven and bake for 15-20 minutes or until the frittata is cooked through.
9. Slice and serve.

Nutritional Information:

Calories: 180 (per serving) | Protein: 12g | Fat: 14g | Net Carbs: 2g | Fiber: 0g

Key Benefits: Eggs provide high-quality protein, mushrooms offer vitamins and minerals, and goat cheese adds a tangy flavor.

Tips: Add sautéed onions or spinach for extra depth of flavor.

15. Cheddar and Broccoli Mini Quiches

Servings: 4-6

Prep Time: 15 minutes

Cook Time: 20 minutes

Ingredients:

- 6 eggs
- 1/2 cup diced cooked broccoli
- 1/2 cup shredded cheddar cheese
- 1/4 cup heavy cream
- Salt and pepper to taste
- Chopped fresh parsley for garnish

Instructions:

1. Preheat the oven to 375°F (190°C) and grease a muffin tin.
2. In a bowl, whisk eggs, heavy cream, salt, and pepper.
3. Divide diced broccoli and shredded cheddar cheese among the muffin cups.
4. Pour the egg mixture into the muffin cups, filling each about 3/4 full.
5. Bake for about 20 minutes or until the quiches are set and slightly golden.
6. Garnish with chopped parsley before serving.

Nutritional Information:

Calories: 180 (per serving) | Protein: 10g | Fat: 14g | Net Carbs: 2g | Fiber: 0g

Key Benefits: Broccoli provides fiber and vitamins, while cheddar cheese adds protein and flavor.

Tips: Add diced ham or bacon for extra protein and flavor.

16. Almond Butter and Berry Smoothie

Servings: 1

Prep Time: 5 minutes

Ingredients:

- 1 cup unsweetened almond milk
- 2 tablespoons almond butter
- 1/4 cup mixed berries (such as strawberries and blueberries)
- 1 scoop low-carb protein powder (optional)
- Ice cubes

Instructions:

1. In a blender, combine almond milk, almond butter, mixed berries, protein powder, and ice cubes.
2. Blend until smooth and creamy.
3. Pour into a glass and enjoy.

Nutritional Information:

Calories: 300 | Protein: 15g | Fat: 23g | Net Carbs: 6g | Fiber: 4g

Key Benefits: Almond butter offers healthy fats and protein, while berries provide antioxidants and vitamins.

Tips: Adjust the sweetness with a touch of low-carb sweetener if desired.

17. Cottage Cheese and Berry Parfait

Servings: 1

Prep Time: 5 minutes

Ingredients:

- 1/2 cup full-fat cottage cheese
- 1/4 cup mixed berries (such as raspberries and blackberries)
- 2 tablespoons chopped nuts (such as almonds or walnuts)
- 1 teaspoon low-carb sweetener (stevia, erythritol, or monk fruit)

Instructions:

1. In a glass or bowl, layer cottage cheese, mixed berries, and chopped nuts.
2. Repeat the layers.
3. Sprinkle the sweetener over the top.
4. Serve immediately.

Nutritional Information:

Calories: 250 | Protein: 15g | Fat: 18g | Net Carbs: 6g | Fiber: 3g

Key Benefits: Cottage cheese provides protein and calcium, while berries offer antioxidants and vitamins.

Tips: Use a flavored cottage cheese for added variety.

18. Chocolate Avocado Smoothie Bowl

Servings: 1

Prep Time: 5 minutes

Ingredients:

- 1 ripe avocado
- 1 cup unsweetened almond milk
- 1 tablespoon unsweetened cocoa powder
- 1 scoop low-carb chocolate protein powder
- 1 teaspoon low-carb sweetener (stevia, erythritol, or monk fruit)
- Toppings: sliced strawberries, shredded coconut, chopped nuts

Instructions:

1. In a blender, combine ripe avocado, almond milk, cocoa powder, protein powder, and sweetener.
2. Blend until smooth and creamy.
3. Pour into a bowl.
4. Top with sliced strawberries, shredded coconut, and chopped nuts.

Nutritional Information:

Calories: 350 | Protein: 15g | Fat: 25g | Net Carbs: 8g | Fiber: 8g

Key Benefits: Avocado offers healthy fats and vitamins, while cocoa powder adds a chocolatey flavor and antioxidants.

Tips: Add a dash of vanilla extract for extra depth of flavor.

19. Cauliflower Breakfast Burrito

Servings: 1

Prep Time: 15 minutes

Cook Time: 10 minutes

Ingredients:

- 2 large collard green leaves
- 1/2 cup cauliflower rice
- 2 eggs, scrambled
- 2 slices cooked turkey bacon, chopped
- 2 tablespoons diced tomatoes
- 2 tablespoons diced red onion
- 2 tablespoons shredded cheddar cheese
- Salt and pepper to taste

Instructions:

1. Wash and trim the stem of the collard green leaves.
2. Blanche the leaves in boiling water for about 30 seconds, then plunge them into ice water to stop the cooking.
3. Lay the leaves flat and pat them dry.
4. In a bowl, mix cauliflower rice with scrambled eggs, chopped turkey bacon, diced tomatoes, diced red onion, and shredded cheddar cheese.
5. Place half of the mixture on each collard green leaf.
6. Fold in the sides of the leaf, then roll it up like a burrito.
7. Slice in half and serve.

Nutritional Information:

Calories: 300 | Protein: 20g | Fat: 18g | Net Carbs: 9g | Fiber: 5g

Key Benefits: Collard green leaves offer a sturdy wrap, while cauliflower rice provides fiber and vitamins.

Tips: Add a dollop of Greek yogurt or sour cream for extra creaminess.

20. Chorizo and Spinach Breakfast Casserole

Servings: 4-6

Prep Time: 15 minutes

Cook Time: 40 minutes

Ingredients:

- 1/2 pound chorizo sausage, cooked and crumbled
- 2 cups fresh spinach
- 1/2 cup diced red bell pepper
- 1/4 cup diced red onion
- 1 cup shredded Monterey Jack cheese
- 6 eggs
- 1/2 cup heavy cream
- Salt and pepper to taste
- Fresh cilantro for garnish

Instructions:

1. Preheat the oven to 375°F (190°C) and grease a baking dish.
2. Spread the cooked chorizo sausage, fresh spinach, diced red bell pepper, and diced red onion in the baking dish.
3. Sprinkle shredded Monterey Jack cheese over the mixture.
4. In a bowl, whisk eggs, heavy cream, salt, and pepper.
5. Pour the egg mixture over the ingredients in the baking dish.

6. Bake for about 35-40 minutes or until the casserole is set and slightly golden.

7. Garnish with fresh cilantro before serving.

Nutritional Information:

Calories: 350 (per serving) | Protein: 20g | Fat: 27g | Net Carbs: 4g | Fiber: 1g

Key Benefits: Chorizo sausage provides flavor and protein, while spinach offers vitamins and minerals.

Tips: Add diced jalapenos for a spicy kick, or substitute chorizo with ground turkey for a leaner option.

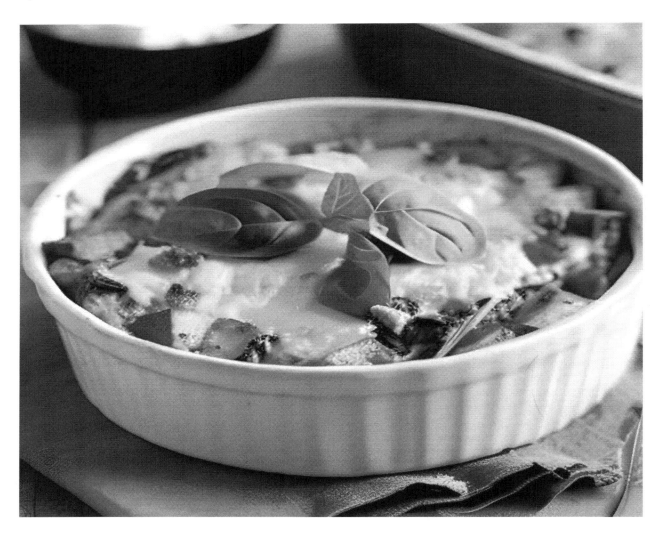

SATISFYING APPETIZERS AND SNACKS

21. Zucchini Fries

Servings: 2-3

Prep Time: 15 minutes

Cook Time: 20 minutes

Ingredients:

- 2 medium zucchinis, cut into fry-sized sticks
- 1/2 cup almond flour
- 1/4 cup grated Parmesan cheese
- 1 teaspoon garlic powder
- Salt and pepper to taste
- 2 eggs, beaten

Instructions:

1. Preheat the oven to 400°F (200°C) and line a baking sheet with parchment paper.
2. In a bowl, mix almond flour, grated Parmesan cheese, garlic powder, salt, and pepper.
3. Dip zucchini sticks in beaten eggs, then coat with the almond flour mixture.
4. Place the coated zucchini sticks on the baking sheet.
5. Bake for about 20 minutes, turning halfway, until the zucchini is golden and crispy.
6. Serve with a low-carb dipping sauce.

Nutritional Information:

Calories: 150 (per serving) | Protein: 8g | Fat: 11g | Net Carbs: 5g | Fiber: 3g

Key Benefits: Zucchini offers vitamins and minerals, while almond flour provides a low-carb coating.

Tips: Add a pinch of cayenne pepper to the coating for a spicy kick.

22. Guacamole Deviled Eggs

Servings: 4-6

Prep Time: 15 minutes

Ingredients:

- 6 hard-boiled eggs, halved
- 1 ripe avocado, mashed
- 2 tablespoons diced red onion
- 1 tablespoon diced tomatoes
- 1 tablespoon chopped fresh cilantro
- Juice of 1 lime
- Salt and pepper to taste
- Paprika for garnish

Instructions:

1. Scoop out the yolks from the halved eggs and place them in a bowl.
2. Mash the yolks with mashed avocado, diced red onion, diced tomatoes, chopped cilantro, lime juice, salt, and pepper.
3. Fill the egg white halves with the guacamole mixture.
4. Sprinkle paprika over the top for color.
5. Serve chilled.

Nutritional Information:

Calories: 150 (per serving) | Protein: 8g | Fat: 11g | Net Carbs: 3g | Fiber: 2g

Key Benefits: Eggs provide protein, while avocado adds healthy fats and vitamins.

Tips: Add diced jalapenos for extra heat, and adjust lime juice to taste.

23. Bacon-Wrapped Asparagus Bundles

Servings: 2-3

Prep Time: 10 minutes

Cook Time: 20 minutes

Ingredients:

- 1 bunch asparagus, trimmed
- 6 slices bacon, cut in half
- 2 tablespoons olive oil
- Salt and pepper to taste

Instructions:

1. Preheat the oven to 400°F (200°C) and line a baking sheet with parchment paper.
2. Toss asparagus with olive oil, salt, and pepper.
3. Bundle 4-5 asparagus spears together and wrap a bacon half around each bundle.
4. Place the bundles on the baking sheet.
5. Bake for about 20 minutes or until the bacon is crispy and the asparagus is tender.
6. Serve as a delightful appetizer or snack.

Nutritional Information:

Calories: 180 (per serving) | Protein: 8g | Fat: 14g | Net Carbs: 2g | Fiber: 2g

Key Benefits: Asparagus provides vitamins and fiber, while bacon offers flavor and healthy fats.

Tips: Drizzle with balsamic reduction for a tangy touch.

24. Cucumber Cream Cheese Bites

Servings: 2-3

Prep Time: 10 minutes

Ingredients:

- 1 cucumber, sliced into rounds
- 1/4 cup cream cheese
- 2 tablespoons diced smoked salmon
- 1 tablespoon chopped fresh dill
- Salt and pepper to taste

Instructions:

1. Spread a thin layer of cream cheese on each cucumber round.
2. Top with diced smoked salmon.
3. Sprinkle chopped dill over the top.
4. Season with salt and pepper.
5. Serve chilled.

Nutritional Information:

Calories: 100 (per serving) | Protein: 5g | Fat: 8g | Net Carbs: 2g | Fiber: 0g

Key Benefits: Cucumber provides hydration and vitamins, while cream cheese and salmon add creaminess and protein.

Tips: Add capers or red onion for extra flavor.

25. Spicy Jalapeno Poppers

Servings: 4-6

Prep Time: 15 minutes

Cook Time: 15 minutes

Ingredients:

- 12 jalapeno peppers, halved and seeds removed
- 1/2 cup cream cheese, softened
- 1/4 cup shredded cheddar cheese
- 1/4 cup cooked and crumbled sausage
- 1 teaspoon garlic powder
- Salt and pepper to taste
- Bacon slices, cooked and crumbled (optional)

Instructions:

1. Preheat the oven to 375°F (190°C) and line a baking sheet with parchment paper.
2. In a bowl, mix cream cheese, shredded cheddar cheese, cooked sausage, garlic powder, salt, and pepper.
3. Fill each jalapeno half with the cream cheese mixture.
4. Place the filled jalapenos on the baking sheet.
5. Bake for about 15 minutes or until the jalapenos are tender and the cheese is melted.
6. Sprinkle with crumbled bacon before serving.

Nutritional Information:

Calories: 150 (per serving) | Protein: 5g | Fat: 12g | Net Carbs: 2g | Fiber: 1g

Key Benefits: Jalapenos provide a spicy kick, while cream cheese and sausage offer protein and flavor.

Tips: Wear gloves when handling jalapenos to avoid skin irritation.

26. Parmesan Crisps with Prosciutto

Servings: 2-3

Prep Time: 5 minutes

Cook Time: 8 minutes

Ingredients:

- 1 cup grated Parmesan cheese
- 6 slices prosciutto

Instructions:

1. Preheat the oven to 400°F (200°C) and line a baking sheet with parchment paper.
2. Spoon small piles of grated Parmesan cheese onto the baking sheet, flattening them slightly.
3. Bake for about 5-8 minutes or until the cheese is melted and golden.
4. Remove from the oven and let cool for a minute to set.
5. Wrap each Parmesan crisp with a slice of prosciutto.
6. Serve as a crunchy and savory snack.

Nutritional Information:

Calories: 200 (per serving) | Protein: 20g | Fat: 12g | Net Carbs: 1g | Fiber: 0g

Key Benefits: Parmesan cheese provides protein and calcium, while prosciutto adds flavor.

Tips: Add a sprinkle of black pepper on the cheese before baking.

27. Tuna Cucumber Bites

Servings: 2-3

Prep Time: 10 minutes

Ingredients:

- 1 cucumber, sliced into rounds
- 1 can tuna, drained
- 2 tablespoons mayonnaise
- 1 tablespoon diced red onion
- 1 tablespoon chopped fresh parsley
- Salt and pepper to taste

Instructions:

1. In a bowl, mix drained tuna with mayonnaise, diced red onion, chopped parsley, salt, and pepper.
2. Spread a spoonful of the tuna mixture onto each cucumber round.
3. Serve chilled.

Nutritional Information:

Calories: 150 (per serving) | Protein: 15g | Fat: 10g | Net Carbs: 2g | Fiber: 0g

Key Benefits: Tuna offers protein and omega-3 fatty acids, while cucumber provides hydration.

Tips: Add a squeeze of lemon juice for a zesty twist.

28. Sausage Stuffed Mushrooms

Servings: 4-6

Prep Time: 15 minutes

Cook Time: 20 minutes

Ingredients:

- 12 large mushrooms, stems removed
- 1/2 pound ground sausage, cooked and crumbled
- 1/4 cup grated Parmesan cheese
- 2 tablespoons chopped fresh parsley
- 1 teaspoon garlic powder
- Salt and pepper to taste

Instructions:

1. Preheat the oven to 375°F (190°C) and line a baking sheet with parchment paper.
2. In a bowl, mix cooked sausage, grated Parmesan cheese, chopped parsley, garlic powder, salt, and pepper.
3. Fill each mushroom cap with the sausage mixture.
4. Place the filled mushrooms on the baking sheet.
5. Bake for about 20 minutes or until the mushrooms are tender and the filling is golden.
6. Serve as a hearty appetizer.

Nutritional Information:

Calories: 150 (per serving) | Protein: 8g | Fat: 12g | Net Carbs: 2g | Fiber: 0g

Key Benefits: Mushrooms offer vitamins and minerals, while sausage provides protein and flavor.

Tips: Sprinkle extra Parmesan cheese on top before baking.

29. Crispy Keto Cheese Chips

Servings: 2-3

Prep Time: 5 minutes

Cook Time: 10 minutes

Ingredients:

- 1 cup shredded cheddar cheese

Instructions:

1. Preheat the oven to 400°F (200°C) and line a baking sheet with parchment paper.
2. Spoon small mounds of shredded cheddar cheese onto the baking sheet, leaving space between them.
3. Gently flatten each mound into a thin circle.
4. Bake for about 6-8 minutes or until the cheese is melted and edges are crispy.
5. Let cool for a minute, then carefully remove the cheese chips from the parchment paper.
6. Serve as a crunchy and satisfying snack.

Nutritional Information:

Calories: 150 (per serving) | Protein: 8g | Fat: 12g | Net Carbs: 1g | Fiber: 0g

Key Benefits: Cheddar cheese provides protein and calcium.

Tips: Add a sprinkle of smoked paprika or cayenne pepper before baking for extra flavor.

30. Cauliflower and Bacon Dip

Servings: 4-6

Prep Time: 15 minutes

Cook Time: 25 minutes

Ingredients:

- 2 cups cauliflower florets
- 4 slices bacon, cooked and crumbled
- 1/2 cup cream cheese
- 1/4 cup shredded cheddar cheese
- 1/4 cup mayonnaise
- 2 tablespoons diced green onions
- 1 teaspoon garlic powder
- Salt and pepper to taste

Instructions:

1. Preheat the oven to 375°F (190°C) and grease a baking dish.
2. Steam cauliflower florets until tender, then chop them into smaller pieces.
3. In a bowl, mix chopped cauliflower, crumbled bacon, cream cheese, shredded cheddar cheese, mayonnaise, diced green onions, garlic powder, salt, and pepper.
4. Spread the mixture evenly in the baking dish.
5. Bake for about 20-25 minutes or until the dip is bubbly and golden on top.
6. Serve with low-carb crackers or vegetable sticks.

Nutritional Information:

Calories: 200 (per serving) | Protein: 8g | Fat: 17g | Net Carbs: 3g | Fiber: 1g

Key Benefits: Cauliflower provides fiber and vitamins, while bacon adds flavor and protein.

Tips: Sprinkle extra shredded cheese on top before baking.

31. Stuffed Bell Pepper Poppers

Servings: 4-6

Prep Time: 15 minutes

Cook Time: 20 minutes

Ingredients:

- 3 large bell peppers, halved and seeds removed
- 1/2 cup cream cheese, softened
- 1/4 cup cooked and crumbled ground beef
- 1/4 cup diced tomatoes
- 1/4 cup shredded Monterey Jack cheese
- 1 teaspoon chili powder
- Salt and pepper to taste

Instructions:

1. Preheat the oven to 375°F (190°C) and line a baking sheet with parchment paper.
2. In a bowl, mix cream cheese, crumbled ground beef, diced tomatoes, shredded Monterey Jack cheese, chili powder, salt, and pepper.
3. Fill each bell pepper half with the cream cheese mixture.
4. Place the filled peppers on the baking sheet.
5. Bake for about 20 minutes or until the peppers are tender and the filling is heated through.
6. Serve as a flavorful appetizer.

Nutritional Information:

Calories: 150 (per serving) | Protein: 8g | Fat: 12g | Net Carbs: 3g | Fiber: 1g

Key Benefits: Bell peppers offer vitamins and antioxidants, while cream cheese and ground beef provide protein and flavor.

Tips: Top with a sprinkle of chopped fresh cilantro before serving.

32. Smoked Salmon Cucumber Bites

Servings: 2-3

Prep Time: 10 minutes

Ingredients:

- 1 cucumber, sliced into rounds
- 4 ounces smoked salmon
- 2 tablespoons cream cheese
- 1 tablespoon capers
- 1 teaspoon chopped fresh dill

Instructions:

1. Spread a thin layer of cream cheese on each cucumber round.
2. Top with a small piece of smoked salmon.
3. Garnish with capers and chopped dill.
4. Serve chilled.

Nutritional Information:

Calories: 150 (per serving) | Protein: 15g | Fat: 8g | Net Carbs: 2g | Fiber: 0g

Key Benefits: Smoked salmon offers protein and omega-3 fatty acids, while cucumber provides hydration.

Tips: Add a squeeze of lemon juice for extra brightness.

33. Spinach and Artichoke Dip Stuffed Mushrooms

Servings: 4-6

Prep Time: 15 minutes

Cook Time: 20 minutes

Ingredients:

- 12 large mushrooms, stems removed
- 1 cup chopped fresh spinach
- 1/2 cup chopped canned artichoke hearts, drained
- 1/4 cup cream cheese
- 1/4 cup shredded mozzarella cheese
- 1/4 cup grated Parmesan cheese
- 1 teaspoon garlic powder
- Salt and pepper to taste

Instructions:

1. Preheat the oven to 375°F (190°C) and line a baking sheet with parchment paper.
2. In a pan, sauté chopped spinach and chopped artichoke hearts until wilted.
3. In a bowl, mix sautéed spinach and artichokes with cream cheese, shredded mozzarella cheese, grated Parmesan cheese, garlic powder, salt, and pepper.
4. Fill each mushroom cap with the spinach and artichoke mixture.
5. Place the filled mushrooms on the baking sheet.
6. Bake for about 20 minutes or until the mushrooms are tender and the filling is bubbly.
7. Serve as a delicious and creamy appetizer.

Nutritional Information:

Calories: 150 (per serving) | Protein: 8g | Fat: 12g | Net Carbs: 2g | Fiber: 1g

Key Benefits: Spinach provides vitamins and minerals, while artichoke hearts add fiber and flavor.

Tips: Add a pinch of red pepper flakes for a touch of heat.

34. Crispy Prosciutto-Wrapped Asparagus

Servings: 2-3

Prep Time: 10 minutes

Cook Time: 15 minutes

Ingredients:

- 12 asparagus spears, trimmed
- 6 slices prosciutto
- Olive oil for drizzling
- Salt and pepper to taste

Instructions:

1. Preheat the oven to 400°F (200°C) and line a baking sheet with parchment paper.
2. Wrap each asparagus spear with a slice of prosciutto, leaving the tips exposed.
3. Place the wrapped asparagus on the baking sheet.
4. Drizzle with olive oil and season with salt and pepper.
5. Bake for about 12-15 minutes or until the prosciutto is crispy and the asparagus is tender.
6. Serve as a flavorful and crunchy appetizer.

Nutritional Information:

Calories: 200 (per serving) | Protein: 15g | Fat: 14g | Net Carbs: 2g | Fiber: 1g

Key Benefits: Asparagus offers vitamins and fiber, while prosciutto adds flavor.

Tips: Sprinkle with grated Parmesan cheese before baking for extra richness.

35. Cottage Cheese Stuffed Bell Peppers

Servings: 2-3

Prep Time: 15 minutes

Ingredients:

- 2 large bell peppers, halved and seeds removed
- 1 cup full-fat cottage cheese
- 1/4 cup diced tomatoes
- 2 tablespoons chopped fresh chives
- 1 tablespoon chopped fresh basil
- Salt and pepper to taste

Instructions:

1. In a bowl, mix cottage cheese, diced tomatoes, chopped chives, chopped basil, salt, and pepper.
2. Fill each bell pepper half with the cottage cheese mixture.
3. Serve chilled as a refreshing and creamy snack.

Nutritional Information:

Calories: 150 (per serving) | Protein: 10g | Fat: 8g | Net Carbs: 4g | Fiber: 1g

Key Benefits: Cottage cheese provides protein and calcium, while bell peppers offer vitamins and antioxidants.

Tips: Add a sprinkle of black pepper on top before serving.

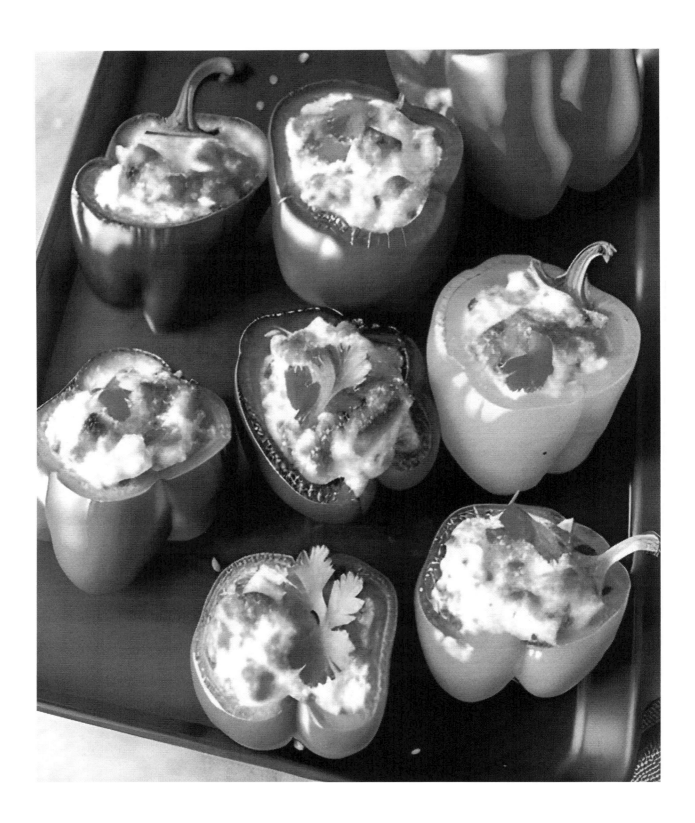

WHOLESOME SOUPS AND SALADS

36. Creamy Broccoli Cheddar Soup

Servings: 4-6

Prep Time: 10 minutes

Cook Time: 25 minutes

Ingredients:

- 2 cups chopped broccoli florets
- 1 small onion, diced
- 2 cloves garlic, minced
- 4 cups chicken or vegetable broth
- 1 cup heavy cream
- 1 cup shredded cheddar cheese
- 2 tablespoons butter
- Salt and pepper to taste

Instructions:

1. In a pot, melt butter and sauté diced onion and minced garlic until fragrant.
2. Add chopped broccoli and cook for a few minutes.
3. Pour in chicken or vegetable broth and bring to a simmer.
4. Let the soup simmer until the broccoli is tender.
5. Use an immersion blender to puree the soup until smooth.
6. Stir in heavy cream and shredded cheddar cheese until melted.
7. Season with salt and pepper.
8. Serve hot.

Nutritional Information:

Calories: 300 (per serving) | Protein: 10g | Fat: 25g | Net Carbs: 5g | Fiber: 2g

Key Benefits: Broccoli provides vitamins and fiber, while cheddar cheese adds creaminess and flavor.

Tips: Garnish with crispy bacon bits or additional shredded cheese.

37. Avocado Cucumber Salad

Servings: 2-3

Prep Time: 10 minutes

Ingredients:

- 2 ripe avocados, diced
- 1 cucumber, diced
- 1/4 cup diced red onion
- 2 tablespoons chopped fresh cilantro
- Juice of 1 lime
- 2 tablespoons olive oil
- Salt and pepper to taste

Instructions:

1. In a bowl, combine diced avocado, diced cucumber, diced red onion, chopped cilantro, lime juice, olive oil, salt, and pepper.
2. Toss gently to combine.
3. Serve as a refreshing and nutritious salad.

Nutritional Information:

Calories: 200 (per serving) | Protein: 2g | Fat: 18g | Net Carbs: 7g | Fiber: 5g

Key Benefits: Avocado offers healthy fats and vitamins, while cucumber provides hydration.

Tips: Add diced tomatoes or bell peppers for extra color and flavor.

38. Spicy Chicken and Kale Soup

Servings: 4-6

Prep Time: 15 minutes

Cook Time: 30 minutes

Ingredients:

- 2 boneless, skinless chicken breasts, diced
- 4 cups chicken broth
- 2 cups chopped kale
- 1 can diced tomatoes
- 1 small onion, diced
- 2 cloves garlic, minced
- 1 teaspoon cumin
- 1 teaspoon chili powder
- 1/2 teaspoon cayenne pepper (adjust to taste)
- Salt and pepper to taste
- Olive oil for cooking

Instructions:

1. In a pot, heat olive oil and sauté diced onion and minced garlic until translucent.

2. Add diced chicken and cook until no longer pink.

3. Stir in cumin, chili powder, cayenne pepper, salt, and pepper.

4. Pour in chicken broth and bring to a boil.

5. Add chopped kale and diced tomatoes, then reduce to a simmer.

6. Let the soup simmer until the kale is tender.

7. Adjust seasoning to taste.

8. Serve hot.

Nutritional Information:

Calories: 250 (per serving) | Protein: 20g | Fat: 10g | Net Carbs: 8g | Fiber: 3g

Key Benefits: Chicken provides protein, while kale offers vitamins and antioxidants.

Tips: Top with a dollop of sour cream for extra creaminess.

39. Grilled Shrimp Salad with Lemon Herb Dressing

Servings: 2-3

Prep Time: 15 minutes

Cook Time: 10 minutes

Ingredients:

- 1 pound large shrimp, peeled and deveined
- 6 cups mixed salad greens
- 1 cup cherry tomatoes, halved
- 1/4 cup sliced red onion
- 1/4 cup crumbled feta cheese
- 2 tablespoons chopped fresh parsley
- Juice of 1 lemon

- 2 tablespoons olive oil
- 1 teaspoon Dijon mustard
- Salt and pepper to taste

Instructions:

1. Preheat a grill or grill pan.
2. Season shrimp with salt and pepper.
3. Grill shrimp for about 2-3 minutes per side or until cooked through.
4. In a bowl, whisk together lemon juice, olive oil, Dijon mustard, salt, and pepper to make the dressing.
5. In a large salad bowl, combine mixed salad greens, halved cherry tomatoes, sliced red onion, crumbled feta cheese, and chopped parsley.
6. Add grilled shrimp on top.
7. Drizzle the lemon herb dressing over the salad.
8. Toss gently to coat.
9. Serve as a satisfying and light salad.

Nutritional Information:

Calories: 300 (per serving) | Protein: 25g | Fat: 15g | Net Carbs: 9g | Fiber: 3g

Key Benefits: Shrimp offers protein and omega-3 fatty acids, while mixed greens provide vitamins and minerals.

Tips: Add sliced avocado for extra creaminess.

40. Cauliflower and Leek Soup

Servings: 4-6

Prep Time: 15 minutes

Cook Time: 25 minutes

Ingredients:

- 1 medium cauliflower head, chopped
- 2 leeks, white and light green parts, sliced
- 4 cups chicken or vegetable broth
- 1 cup heavy cream
- 2 tablespoons butter
- Salt and pepper to taste
- Chopped fresh chives for garnish

Instructions:

1. In a pot, melt butter and sauté sliced leeks until tender.
2. Add chopped cauliflower and cook for a few minutes.
3. Pour in chicken or vegetable broth and bring to a simmer.
4. Let the soup simmer until the cauliflower is tender.
5. Use an immersion blender to puree the soup until smooth.
6. Stir in heavy cream and season with salt and pepper.
7. Serve hot, garnished with chopped chives.

Nutritional Information:

Calories: 250 (per serving) | Protein: 5g | Fat: 20g | Net Carbs: 7g | Fiber: 2g

Key Benefits: Cauliflower provides fiber and vitamins, while leeks add flavor and antioxidants.

Tips: Top with grated Parmesan cheese or crispy bacon bits.

41. Greek Salad with Grilled Chicken

Servings: 2-3

Prep Time: 15 minutes

Cook Time: 15 minutes

Ingredients:

- 2 boneless, skinless chicken breasts
- 6 cups mixed salad greens
- 1 cup cucumber, diced
- 1 cup cherry tomatoes, halved
- 1/4 cup sliced red onion
- 1/4 cup crumbled feta cheese
- 2 tablespoons chopped fresh oregano
- 2 tablespoons olive oil
- Juice of 1 lemon
- Salt and pepper to taste

Instructions:

1. Preheat a grill or grill pan.
2. Season chicken breasts with chopped fresh oregano, olive oil, salt, and pepper.
3. Grill chicken for about 6-7 minutes per side or until cooked through.
4. Slice grilled chicken into strips.
5. In a large salad bowl, combine mixed salad greens, diced cucumber, halved cherry tomatoes, sliced red onion, and crumbled feta cheese.
6. Add sliced grilled chicken on top.
7. Drizzle with olive oil and lemon juice.
8. Toss gently to combine.
9. Serve as a Mediterranean-inspired salad.

Nutritional Information:

Calories: 300 (per serving) | Protein: 25g | Fat: 15g | Net Carbs: 8g | Fiber: 3g

Key Benefits: Grilled chicken provides protein, while mixed greens offer vitamins and minerals.

Tips: Add Kalamata olives for extra Greek flair.

42. Mexican Cauliflower Rice Salad

Servings: 4-6

Prep Time: 15 minutes

Ingredients:

4 cups cauliflower rice (fresh or frozen)

- 1 can black beans, drained and rinsed
- 1 cup diced bell peppers
- 1/2 cup diced red onion
- 1/4 cup chopped fresh cilantro
- Juice of 1 lime
- 2 tablespoons olive oil
- 1 teaspoon cumin
- 1 teaspoon chili powder
- Salt and pepper to taste

Instructions:

1. In a bowl, mix cauliflower rice, black beans, diced bell peppers, diced red onion, chopped cilantro, lime juice, olive oil, cumin, chili powder, salt, and pepper.
2. Toss gently to combine.

3. Serve as a flavorful and low-carb salad.

Nutritional Information:

Calories: 200 (per serving) | Protein: 8g | Fat: 10g | Net Carbs: 7g | Fiber: 3g

Key Benefits: Cauliflower rice offers a low-carb base, while black beans provide protein and fiber.

Tips: Top with diced avocado or a dollop of Greek yogurt.

43. Tomato Basil Soup with Parmesan Crisps

Servings: 4-6

Prep Time: 10 minutes

Cook Time: 25 minutes

Ingredients:

- 4 cups diced tomatoes (canned or fresh)
- 2 cups chicken or vegetable broth
- 1/2 cup heavy cream
- 1/4 cup chopped fresh basil
- 2 cloves garlic, minced
- 1 small onion, diced
- 2 tablespoons olive oil
- Salt and pepper to taste
- Grated Parmesan cheese for garnish

Instructions:

1. In a pot, heat olive oil and sauté diced onion and minced garlic until translucent.
2. Add diced tomatoes and cook for a few minutes.

3. Pour in chicken or vegetable broth and bring to a simmer.

4. Let the soup simmer for about 15-20 minutes.

5. Use an immersion blender to puree the soup until smooth.

6. Stir in heavy cream and chopped fresh basil.

7. Season with salt and pepper.

8. Serve hot, garnished with grated Parmesan cheese.

Nutritional Information:

Calories: 250 (per serving) | Protein: 5g | Fat: 20g | Net Carbs: 9g | Fiber: 2g

Key Benefits: Tomatoes provide vitamins and antioxidants, while basil adds fresh flavor.

Tips: Serve with homemade Parmesan crisps for added crunch.

44. Asian Cabbage Salad with Grilled Steak

Servings: 2-3

Prep Time: 20 minutes

Cook Time: 10 minutes

Ingredients:

- 1 pound steak (such as flank or sirloin)
- 6 cups shredded cabbage
- 1 cup shredded carrots
- 1/4 cup sliced green onions
- 1/4 cup chopped fresh cilantro
- 2 tablespoons sesame oil
- 2 tablespoons soy sauce (or tamari for gluten-free)
- 1 tablespoon rice vinegar

- 1 teaspoon grated fresh ginger
- Salt and pepper to taste

Instructions:

- Preheat a grill or grill pan.
- Season steak with salt and pepper.
- Grill steak for about 4-5 minutes per side for medium-rare, or until desired doneness.
- Let the steak rest before slicing.
- In a large bowl, combine shredded cabbage, shredded carrots, sliced green onions, and chopped cilantro.
- In a small bowl, whisk together sesame oil, soy sauce, rice vinegar, grated fresh ginger, salt, and pepper to make the dressing.
- Add sliced grilled steak on top of the salad.
- Drizzle the dressing over the salad.
- Toss gently to coat.
- Serve as an Asian-inspired and satisfying salad.

Nutritional Information:

Calories: 350 (per serving) | Protein: 30g | Fat: 20g | Net Carbs: 9g | Fiber: 4g

Key Benefits: Grilled steak provides protein, while cabbage and carrots offer vitamins and fiber.

Tips: Top with toasted sesame seeds for added crunch.

45. Creamy Mushroom Soup

Servings: 4-6

Prep Time: 10 minutes

Cook Time: 25 minutes

Ingredients:

- 2 cups sliced mushrooms
- 1 small onion, diced
- 2 cloves garlic, minced
- 4 cups chicken or vegetable broth
- 1 cup heavy cream
- 2 tablespoons butter
- 2 tablespoons chopped fresh thyme
- Salt and pepper to taste

Instructions:

1. In a pot, melt butter and sauté diced onion and minced garlic until translucent.
2. Add sliced mushrooms and cook until browned.
3. Pour in chicken or vegetable broth and bring to a simmer.
4. Let the soup simmer for about 15-20 minutes.
5. Use an immersion blender to puree the soup until smooth.
6. Stir in heavy cream and chopped fresh thyme.
7. Season with salt and pepper.
8. Serve hot.

Nutritional Information:

Calories: 300 (per serving) | Protein: 5g | Fat: 25g | Net Carbs: 7g | Fiber: 1g

Key Benefits: Mushrooms provide vitamins and minerals, while thyme adds flavor and antioxidants.

Tips: Garnish with a drizzle of truffle oil for a luxurious touch.

46. Cobb Salad with Ranch Dressing

Servings: 2-3

Prep Time: 15 minutes

Ingredients:

- 2 cups cooked and diced chicken breast
- 6 cups mixed salad greens
- 1 cup diced cucumber
- 1/2 cup crumbled blue cheese
- 1/4 cup diced tomatoes
- 1/4 cup diced cooked bacon
- 2 hard-boiled eggs, sliced
- 1/4 cup diced red onion
- 2 tablespoons chopped fresh chives
- Salt and pepper to taste
- Ranch dressing for drizzling

Instructions:

1. In a large salad bowl, combine diced cooked chicken breast, mixed salad greens, diced cucumber, crumbled blue cheese, diced tomatoes, diced cooked bacon, sliced hard-boiled eggs, diced red onion, and chopped fresh chives.
2. Drizzle with ranch dressing.
3. Toss gently to combine.

4. Serve as a hearty and flavorful salad.

Nutritional Information:

Calories: 350 (per serving) | Protein: 25g | Fat: 20g | Net Carbs: 9g | Fiber: 3g

Key Benefits: Chicken provides protein, while blue cheese adds richness and flavor.

Tips: Substitute turkey bacon for a leaner option.

47. Roasted Red Pepper and Tomato Soup

Servings: 4-6

Prep Time: 15 minutes

Cook Time: 30 minutes

Ingredients:

- 2 red bell peppers, roasted and peeled
- 4 cups diced tomatoes (canned or fresh)
- 1 small onion, diced
- 2 cloves garlic, minced
- 4 cups chicken or vegetable broth
- 1/2 cup heavy cream
- 2 tablespoons olive oil
- Salt and pepper to taste
- Fresh basil leaves for garnish

Instructions:

1. Preheat the oven to 400°F (200°C).
2. Place red bell peppers on a baking sheet and roast in the oven until the skin is charred.

3. Remove the peppers from the oven and place them in a bowl covered with plastic wrap. This will make it easier to peel the skin.

4. Once cooled, peel the skin off the peppers and dice them.

5. In a pot, heat olive oil and sauté diced onion and minced garlic until translucent.

6. Add diced tomatoes and diced roasted red peppers, and cook for a few minutes.

7. Pour in chicken or vegetable broth and bring to a simmer.

8. Let the soup simmer for about 15-20 minutes.

9. Use an immersion blender to puree the soup until smooth.

10. Stir in heavy cream and season with salt and pepper.

11. Serve hot, garnished with fresh basil leaves.

Nutritional Information:

Calories: 250 (per serving) | Protein: 5g | Fat: 20g | Net Carbs: 9g | Fiber: 2g

Key Benefits: Red bell peppers provide vitamins and antioxidants, while tomatoes add rich flavor.

Tips: Top with a drizzle of balsamic reduction for extra sweetness.

48. Spinach and Strawberry Salad

Servings: 2-3

Prep Time: 10 minutes

Ingredients:

- 6 cups baby spinach leaves
- 1 cup sliced strawberries
- 1/4 cup crumbled goat cheese
- 1/4 cup chopped walnuts
- 2 tablespoons balsamic vinegar
- 2 tablespoons olive oil
- 1 teaspoon honey (optional)
- Salt and pepper to taste

Instructions:

1. In a large salad bowl, combine baby spinach leaves, sliced strawberries, crumbled goat cheese, and chopped walnuts.
2. In a small bowl, whisk together balsamic vinegar, olive oil, honey (if using), salt, and pepper to make the dressing.
3. Drizzle the dressing over the salad.
4. Toss gently to combine.
5. Serve as a sweet and savory salad.

Nutritional Information:

Calories: 250 (per serving) | Protein: 5g | Fat: 20g | Net Carbs: 9g | Fiber: 3g

Key Benefits: Spinach offers vitamins and antioxidants, while strawberries add natural sweetness.

Tips: Substitute honey with a low-carb sweetener for a keto-friendly version.

49. Lemon Chicken Orzo Soup

Servings: 4-6

Prep Time: 15 minutes

Cook Time: 25 minutes

Ingredients:

- 2 cups diced cooked chicken breast
- 1 cup orzo pasta
- 4 cups chicken broth
- 2 cups chopped spinach leaves
- Juice of 2 lemons
- 2 cloves garlic, minced
- 1 small onion, diced
- 2 tablespoons olive oil
- Salt and pepper to taste
- Chopped fresh parsley for garnish

Instructions:

1. In a pot, heat olive oil and sauté diced onion and minced garlic until translucent.
2. Add orzo pasta and cook for a few minutes.
3. Pour in chicken broth and bring to a boil.
4. Let the soup simmer for about 10-12 minutes or until the orzo is cooked.
5. Stir in diced cooked chicken breast, chopped spinach leaves, and lemon juice.
6. Season with salt and pepper.
7. Serve hot, garnished with chopped fresh parsley.

Nutritional Information:

Calories: 300 (per serving) | Protein: 20g | Fat: 10g | Net Carbs: 8g | Fiber: 2g

Key Benefits: Chicken provides protein, while spinach offers vitamins and minerals.

Tips: Add a sprinkle of grated Parmesan cheese before serving.

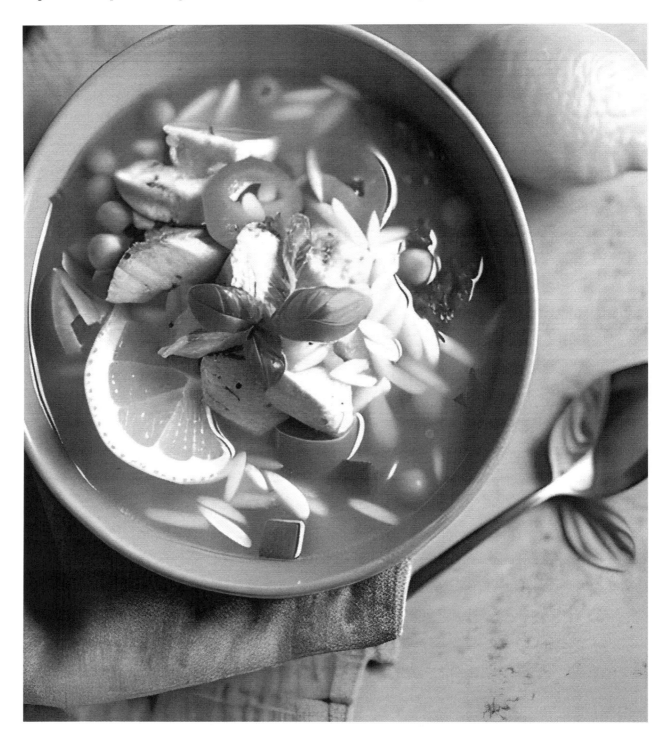

50. Zucchini Noodle Salad with Pesto Dressing

Servings: 2-3

Prep Time: 15 minutes

Ingredients:

- 2 large zucchinis, spiralized into noodles
- 1 cup cherry tomatoes, halved
- 1/4 cup crumbled feta cheese
- 1/4 cup chopped fresh basil
- 1/4 cup chopped walnuts
- 2 tablespoons olive oil
- 2 tablespoons pesto sauce
- Juice of 1 lemon
- Salt and pepper to taste

Instructions:

1. In a bowl, combine zucchini noodle strands, halved cherry tomatoes, crumbled feta cheese, chopped fresh basil, and chopped walnuts.
2. In a small bowl, whisk together olive oil, pesto sauce, lemon juice, salt, and pepper to make the dressing.
3. Drizzle the dressing over the salad.
4. Toss gently to combine.
5. Serve as a light and flavorful salad.

Nutritional Information:

Calories: 250 (per serving) | Protein: 5g | Fat: 20g | Net Carbs: 7g | Fiber: 3g

Key Benefits: Zucchini noodles provide a low-carb base, while pesto adds vibrant flavor.

Tips: Add grilled chicken or shrimp for extra protein.

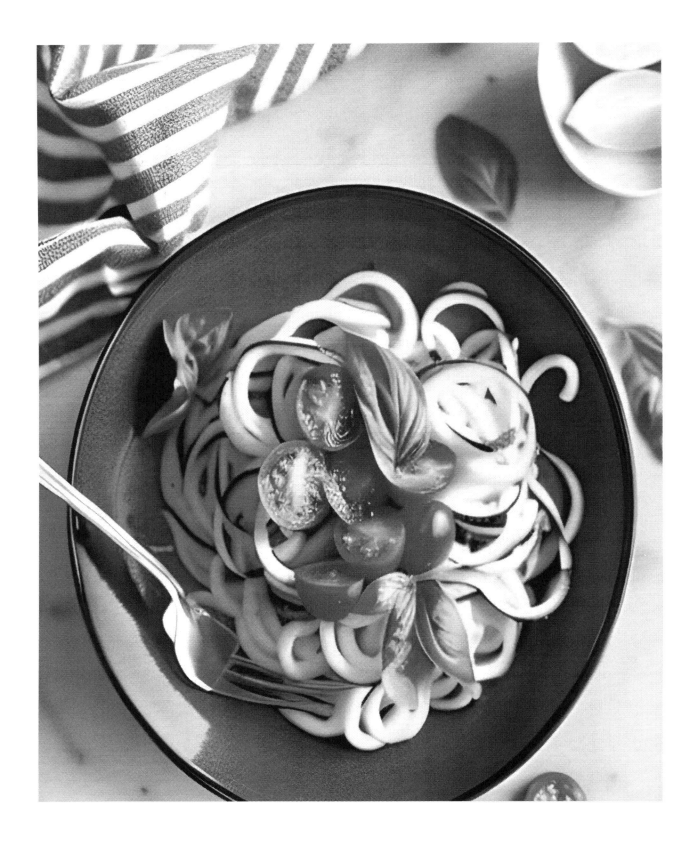

FLAVORFUL POULTRY AND MEAT DISHES

51. Lemon Herb Grilled Chicken

Servings: 2-3

Prep Time: 15 minutes

Cook Time: 15 minutes

Ingredients:

- 2 boneless, skinless chicken breasts
- Juice of 2 lemons
- 2 cloves garlic, minced
- 2 tablespoons chopped fresh rosemary
- 2 tablespoons olive oil
- Salt and pepper to taste

Instructions:

1. In a bowl, combine lemon juice, minced garlic, chopped fresh rosemary, olive oil, salt, and pepper to make the marinade.
2. Place chicken breasts in the marinade and let them marinate for at least 30 minutes.
3. Preheat a grill or grill pan.
4. Grill chicken for about 6-7 minutes per side or until cooked through.
5. Serve hot with a side of steamed vegetables.

Nutritional Information:

Calories: 300 (per serving) | Protein: 25g | Fat: 15g | Net Carbs: 2g | Fiber: 0g

Key Benefits: Chicken provides lean protein, while lemon and rosemary add fresh flavor.

Tips: Substitute chicken thighs for a slightly higher fat content.

52. Spicy Cajun Shrimp Skewers

Servings: 2-3

Prep Time: 10 minutes

Cook Time: 5 minutes

Ingredients:

- 1 pound large shrimp, peeled and deveined
- 2 tablespoons Cajun seasoning
- 2 tablespoons olive oil
- Juice of 1 lime
- Salt and pepper to taste

Instructions:

1. In a bowl, combine Cajun seasoning, olive oil, lime juice, salt, and pepper to make the marinade.
2. Toss shrimp in the marinade and let them marinate for about 15 minutes.
3. Preheat a grill or grill pan.
4. Thread marinated shrimp onto skewers.
5. Grill shrimp skewers for about 2-3 minutes per side or until cooked through.
6. Serve hot with a side of coleslaw.

Nutritional Information:

Calories: 250 (per serving) | Protein: 20g | Fat: 15g | Net Carbs: 2g | Fiber: 0g

Key Benefits: Shrimp offers protein and omega-3 fatty acids, while Cajun seasoning adds bold flavor.

Tips: Serve with a squeeze of fresh lemon for added zing.

53. Garlic Butter Steak Bites

Servings: 2-3

Prep Time: 10 minutes

Cook Time: 10 minutes

Ingredients:

- 1 pound sirloin steak, cut into bite-sized pieces
- 4 tablespoons unsalted butter
- 4 cloves garlic, minced
- 2 tablespoons chopped fresh parsley
- Salt and pepper to taste

Instructions:

1. In a skillet, melt butter over medium heat.
2. Add minced garlic and sauté until fragrant.
3. Add steak bites and cook for about 2-3 minutes per side for medium-rare, or until desired doneness.
4. Stir in chopped fresh parsley, salt, and pepper.
5. Serve hot with a side salad.

Nutritional Information:

Calories: 350 (per serving) | Protein: 25g | Fat: 25g | Net Carbs: 1g | Fiber: 0g

Key Benefits: Steak provides protein and iron, while garlic butter adds rich flavor.

Tips: Top with grated Parmesan cheese for extra umami.

54. Baked Mediterranean Chicken Thighs

Servings: 2-3

Prep Time: 10 minutes

Cook Time: 30 minutes

Ingredients:

- 4 bone-in, skin-on chicken thighs
- 1/4 cup chopped Kalamata olives
- 1/4 cup diced cherry tomatoes
- 1/4 cup crumbled feta cheese
- 2 tablespoons chopped fresh oregano
- 2 tablespoons olive oil
- Juice of 1 lemon
- Salt and pepper to taste

Instructions:

1. Preheat the oven to 375°F (190°C).
2. In a bowl, combine chopped Kalamata olives, diced cherry tomatoes, crumbled feta cheese, chopped fresh oregano, olive oil, lemon juice, salt, and pepper to make the topping.
3. Place chicken thighs in a baking dish.
4. Spread the olive and tomato topping over the chicken.
5. Bake for about 25-30 minutes or until the chicken is cooked through and the skin is crispy.
6. Serve hot with a side of cauliflower rice.

Nutritional Information:

Calories: 400 (per serving) | Protein: 30g | Fat: 30g | Net Carbs: 3g | Fiber: 1g

Key Benefits: Chicken thighs offer flavorful and juicy meat, while Mediterranean toppings add tangy and fresh notes.

Tips: Use boneless, skinless chicken thighs for a lighter option.

55. Stuffed Portobello Mushrooms with Ground Turkey

Servings: 2-3

Prep Time: 15 minutes

Cook Time: 25 minutes

Ingredients:

- 4 large Portobello mushrooms, stems removed
- 1/2 pound ground turkey
- 1/2 cup diced bell peppers
- 1/4 cup diced onion
- 2 cloves garlic, minced
- 1/4 cup shredded mozzarella cheese
- 2 tablespoons chopped fresh parsley
- 2 tablespoons olive oil
- Salt and pepper to taste

Instructions:

1. Preheat the oven to 375°F (190°C).

2. In a skillet, heat olive oil and sauté diced bell peppers, diced onion, and minced garlic until softened.

3. Add ground turkey and cook until browned and cooked through.

4. Stir in chopped fresh parsley, salt, and pepper.

5. Place Portobello mushrooms on a baking sheet.

6. Divide the ground turkey mixture among the mushrooms.

7. Top with shredded mozzarella cheese.

8. Bake for about 20-25 minutes or until the mushrooms are tender and the cheese is melted.

9. Serve hot with a side salad.

Nutritional Information:

Calories: 350 (per serving) | Protein: 25g | Fat: 20g | Net Carbs: 6g | Fiber: 2g

Key Benefits: Ground turkey provides lean protein, while Portobello mushrooms offer a meaty and earthy base.

Tips: Substitute ground chicken or beef if desired.

56. Thai Basil Ground Pork Stir-Fry

Servings: 2-3

Prep Time: 10 minutes

Cook Time: 15 minutes

Ingredients:

- 1/2 pound ground pork
- 1 cup diced bell peppers
- 1/2 cup diced onion
- 2 cloves garlic, minced

- 2 tablespoons chopped fresh Thai basil leaves
- 2 tablespoons fish sauce
- 1 tablespoon soy sauce (or tamari for gluten-free)
- 1 tablespoon olive oil
- Red pepper flakes (optional, for extra heat)
- Salt and pepper to taste

Instructions:

1. In a skillet, heat olive oil and sauté diced bell peppers, diced onion, and minced garlic until softened.
2. Add ground pork and cook until browned and cooked through.
3. Stir in fish sauce, soy sauce, chopped fresh Thai basil leaves, red pepper flakes (if using), salt, and pepper.
4. Cook for another 2-3 minutes to meld the flavors.
5. Serve hot over cauliflower rice.

Nutritional Information:

Calories: 300 (per serving) | Protein: 20g | Fat: 20g | Net Carbs: 4g | Fiber: 1g

Key Benefits: Ground pork offers protein and flavor, while Thai basil leaves add aromatic notes.

Tips: Top with chopped peanuts for extra crunch.

57. Italian Meatball Zoodle Bowl

Servings: 2-3

Prep Time: 20 minutes

Cook Time: 25 minutes

Ingredients:

- 1/2 pound ground beef
- 1/2 cup grated Parmesan cheese
- 1/4 cup chopped fresh parsley
- 2 cloves garlic, minced
- 1 egg
- 2 zucchinis, spiralized into zoodles
- 1 cup marinara sauce (sugar-free)
- 2 tablespoons olive oil
- Salt and pepper to taste

Instructions:

1. Preheat the oven to 375°F (190°C).
2. In a bowl, combine ground beef, grated Parmesan cheese, chopped fresh parsley, minced garlic, and egg to make the meatball mixture.
3. Form the mixture into meatballs and place them on a baking sheet.
4. Bake meatballs for about 20-25 minutes or until cooked through.
5. In a skillet, heat olive oil and sauté zucchini zoodles until tender.
6. Warm marinara sauce in a separate pan.
7. Serve meatballs over zoodles with marinara sauce.

Nutritional Information:

Calories: 350 (per serving) | Protein: 25g | Fat: 25g | Net Carbs: 5g | Fiber: 2g

Key Benefits: Ground beef provides protein and iron, while zucchini zoodles offer a low-carb pasta alternative.

Tips: Use ground turkey or chicken for a leaner option.

58. Smoky BBQ Pulled Pork Lettuce Wraps

Servings: 2-3

Prep Time: 15 minutes

Cook Time: 6 hours (slow cooker)

Ingredients:

- 1 pound pork shoulder or butt roast
- 1 cup sugar-free BBQ sauce
- 1/2 cup chicken broth
- 2 tablespoons smoked paprika
- 2 tablespoons apple cider vinegar
- 1 tablespoon olive oil
- Lettuce leaves (such as iceberg or butter lettuce) for wrapping
- Salt and pepper to taste

Instructions:

1. In a slow cooker, combine chicken broth, smoked paprika, apple cider vinegar, salt, and pepper.
2. Place pork shoulder or butt roast in the slow cooker and cook on low for about 6 hours or until the pork is tender and can be easily shredded.
3. Once cooked, shred the pork using two forks.

4. Mix in sugar-free BBQ sauce to the shredded pork.

5. Heat olive oil in a skillet and warm the BBQ pork mixture.

6. Serve the smoky pulled pork in lettuce leaves for wraps.

Nutritional Information:

Calories: 350 (per serving) | Protein: 25g | Fat: 20g | Net Carbs: 6g | Fiber: 1g

Key Benefits: Pork offers protein, while sugar-free BBQ sauce adds smoky and tangy flavor.

Tips: Top with sliced red onion and chopped pickles for extra crunch and flavor.

59. Mushroom and Swiss Stuffed Chicken Breast

Servings: 2-3

Prep Time: 15 minutes

Cook Time: 25 minutes

Ingredients:

- 2 boneless, skinless chicken breasts
- 1 cup sliced mushrooms
- 1/2 cup shredded Swiss cheese
- 2 tablespoons chopped fresh thyme
- 2 tablespoons butter
- Salt and pepper to taste

Instructions:

1. Preheat the oven to 375°F (190°C).

2. In a skillet, melt butter and sauté sliced mushrooms until browned.

3. Stir in chopped fresh thyme, salt, and pepper.

4. Make a horizontal slit in each chicken breast to create a pocket.

5. Stuff each chicken breast with sautéed mushrooms and shredded Swiss cheese.

6. Secure the openings with toothpicks.

7. Place stuffed chicken breasts in a baking dish.

8. Bake for about 20-25 minutes or until the chicken is cooked through.

9. Serve hot with a side of steamed vegetables.

Nutritional Information:

Calories: 350 (per serving) | Protein: 30g | Fat: 20g | Net Carbs: 2g | Fiber: 0g

Key Benefits: Chicken provides protein, while mushrooms add an earthy and savory touch.

Tips: Substitute Swiss cheese with mozzarella or cheddar if desired.

60. Greek Lamb Souvlaki

Servings: 2-3

Prep Time: 20 minutes

Cook Time: 10 minutes

Ingredients:

- 1/2 pound lamb leg or shoulder, cut into bite-sized pieces
- 1/4 cup olive oil
- 2 tablespoons lemon juice
- 2 cloves garlic, minced
- 1 teaspoon dried oregano
- 1/2 teaspoon ground cumin
- Salt and pepper to taste

Instructions:

1. In a bowl, combine olive oil, lemon juice, minced garlic, dried oregano, ground cumin, salt, and pepper to make the marinade.
2. Add lamb pieces to the marinade and let them marinate for at least 1 hour.
3. Preheat a grill or grill pan.
4. Thread marinated lamb pieces onto skewers.
5. Grill lamb souvlaki for about 3-4 minutes per side or until cooked to your desired level of doneness.
6. Serve hot with a side of Greek salad.

Nutritional Information:

Calories: 300 (per serving) | Protein: 20g | Fat: 25g | Net Carbs: 1g | Fiber: 0g

Key Benefits: Lamb offers protein and essential nutrients, while Greek-inspired flavors add zest.

Tips: Serve with a dollop of tzatziki sauce for extra creaminess.

DELICIOUS SEAFOOD RECIPES

61. Lemon Herb Baked Salmon

Servings: 2-3

Prep Time: 10 minutes

Cook Time: 15 minutes

Ingredients:

- 2 salmon fillets (6-8 ounces each)
- Juice of 1 lemon
- 2 tablespoons chopped fresh dill
- 2 tablespoons olive oil
- Salt and pepper to taste

Instructions:

1. Preheat the oven to 375°F (190°C).
2. Place salmon fillets on a baking sheet.
3. In a bowl, combine lemon juice, chopped fresh dill, olive oil, salt, and pepper to make the marinade.
4. Brush the marinade over the salmon fillets.
5. Bake for about 12-15 minutes or until the salmon flakes easily with a fork.
6. Serve hot with a side of steamed asparagus.

Nutritional Information:

Calories: 300 (per serving) | Protein: 25g | Fat: 20g | Net Carbs: 2g | Fiber: 0g

Key Benefits: Salmon is rich in omega-3 fatty acids, while lemon and dill add vibrant flavor.

Tips: Try different herbs such as thyme or rosemary for variety.

62. Coconut Shrimp Curry

Servings: 2-3

Prep Time: 15 minutes

Cook Time: 20 minutes

Ingredients:

- 1 pound large shrimp, peeled and deveined
- 1 can (14 ounces) coconut milk
- 1 tablespoon red curry paste
- 1 tablespoon fish sauce
- 1 tablespoon olive oil
- 1 red bell pepper, sliced
- 1 zucchini, sliced
- 1 tablespoon chopped fresh cilantro
- Salt and pepper to taste

Instructions:

1. In a skillet, heat olive oil and sauté sliced red bell pepper and sliced zucchini until softened.
2. Stir in red curry paste and cook for a minute.
3. Pour in coconut milk and fish sauce.
4. Add shrimp and let them cook for about 5-7 minutes or until pink and cooked through.
5. Season with salt and pepper.
6. Serve hot, garnished with chopped fresh cilantro.

Nutritional Information:

Calories: 350 (per serving) | Protein: 20g | Fat: 25g | Net Carbs: 5g | Fiber: 1g

Key Benefits: Shrimp offers protein and omega-3 fatty acids, while coconut milk adds creaminess.

Tips: Adjust the amount of curry paste for desired spice level.

63. Lime Cilantro Grilled Swordfish

Servings: 2-3

Prep Time: 10 minutes

Cook Time: 10 minutes

Ingredients:

- 2 swordfish steaks (6-8 ounces each)
- Juice of 2 limes
- 2 tablespoons chopped fresh cilantro
- 2 tablespoons olive oil
- 1 teaspoon ground cumin
- Salt and pepper to taste

Instructions:

1. Preheat a grill or grill pan.
2. In a bowl, combine lime juice, chopped fresh cilantro, olive oil, ground cumin, salt, and pepper to make the marinade.
3. Brush the marinade over swordfish steaks.
4. Grill swordfish for about 4-5 minutes per side or until cooked through and flakes easily.
5. Serve hot with a side of sautéed spinach.

Nutritional Information:

Calories: 300 (per serving) | Protein: 25g | Fat: 20g | Net Carbs: 2g | Fiber: 0g

Key Benefits: Swordfish offers protein and healthy fats, while lime and cilantro add zesty flavor.

Tips: Serve over cauliflower rice for a complete meal.

64. Spicy Garlic Butter Shrimp Skillet

Servings: 2-3

Prep Time: 10 minutes

Cook Time: 10 minutes

Ingredients:

- 1 pound large shrimp, peeled and deveined
- 4 tablespoons unsalted butter
- 4 cloves garlic, minced
- 1 teaspoon red pepper flakes (adjust to taste)
- 1 teaspoon paprika
- Juice of 1 lemon
- Salt and pepper to taste

Instructions:

1. In a skillet, melt butter over medium heat.
2. Add minced garlic and sauté until fragrant.
3. Stir in red pepper flakes and paprika.
4. Add shrimp and cook for about 2-3 minutes per side or until pink and cooked through.
5. Squeeze lemon juice over the shrimp.

6. Season with salt and pepper.

7. Serve hot, garnished with chopped fresh parsley.

Nutritional Information:

Calories: 300 (per serving) | Protein: 20g | Fat: 20g | Net Carbs: 2g | Fiber: 0g

Key Benefits: Shrimp offers protein and omega-3 fatty acids, while garlic butter adds rich flavor.

Tips: Adjust the amount of red pepper flakes for desired spiciness.

65. Sesame Ginger Glazed Salmon

Servings: 2-3

Prep Time: 15 minutes

Cook Time: 15 minutes

Ingredients:

- 2 salmon fillets (6-8 ounces each)
- 2 tablespoons low-sodium soy sauce (or tamari for gluten-free)
- 1 tablespoon olive oil
- 1 tablespoon grated fresh ginger
- 1 tablespoon sesame oil
- 1 tablespoon rice vinegar
- 1 tablespoon sesame seeds
- Salt and pepper to taste

Instructions:

1. Preheat the oven to 375°F (190°C).

2. In a bowl, combine low-sodium soy sauce, olive oil, grated fresh ginger, sesame oil, rice vinegar, salt, and pepper to make the glaze.

3. Brush the glaze over salmon fillets.

4. Sprinkle sesame seeds over the glaze.

5. Bake for about 12-15 minutes or until the salmon flakes easily with a fork.

6. Serve hot with a side of stir-fried bok choy.

Nutritional Information:

Calories: 300 (per serving) | Protein: 25g | Fat: 20g | Net Carbs: 2g | Fiber: 0g

Key Benefits: Salmon is rich in omega-3 fatty acids, while ginger and sesame add depth of flavor.

Tips: Drizzle extra glaze over the bok choy for extra flavor.

66. Garlic Lemon Butter Scallops

Servings: 2-3

Prep Time: 10 minutes

Cook Time: 5 minutes

Ingredients:

- 1 pound sea scallops
- 4 tablespoons unsalted butter
- 4 cloves garlic, minced
- Juice of 1 lemon
- 1 tablespoon chopped fresh parsley
- Salt and pepper to taste

Instructions:

1. In a skillet, melt butter over medium heat.
2. Add minced garlic and sauté until fragrant.
3. Add sea scallops and cook for about 1-2 minutes per side or until they are golden brown and cooked through.
4. Squeeze lemon juice over the scallops.
5. Season with salt and pepper.
6. Serve hot, garnished with chopped fresh parsley.

Nutritional Information:

Calories: 300 (per serving) | Protein: 20g | Fat: 20g | Net Carbs: 2g | Fiber: 0g

Key Benefits: Scallops offer protein and are a good source of vitamin B12, while garlic lemon butter adds rich flavor.

Tips: Serve over cauliflower rice or zucchini noodles.

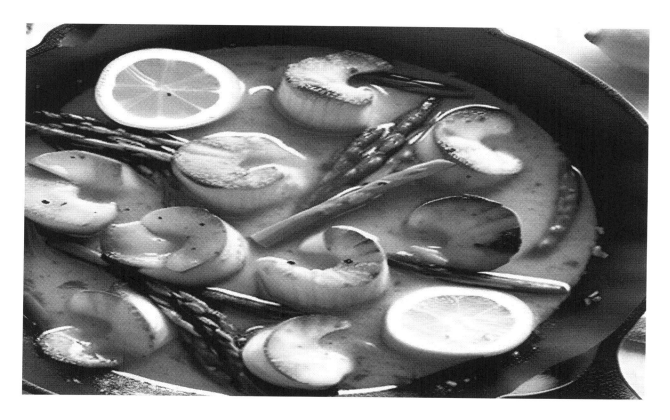

67. Cajun Grilled Catfish

Servings: 2-3

Prep Time: 10 minutes

Cook Time: 10 minutes

Ingredients:

- 2 catfish fillets (6-8 ounces each)
- 1 tablespoon Cajun seasoning
- 2 tablespoons olive oil
- Juice of 1 lime
- Salt and pepper to taste

Instructions:

1. Preheat a grill or grill pan.
2. In a bowl, combine Cajun seasoning, olive oil, lime juice, salt, and pepper to make the marinade.
3. Brush the marinade over catfish fillets.
4. Grill catfish for about 4-5 minutes per side or until cooked through and flakes easily.
5. Serve hot with a side of coleslaw.

Nutritional Information:

Calories: 250 (per serving) | Protein: 20g | Fat: 15g | Net Carbs: 1g | Fiber: 0g

Key Benefits: Catfish offers protein and is low in calories, while Cajun seasoning adds bold flavor.

Tips: Serve with a squeeze of fresh lemon for extra zest.

68. Miso Glazed Cod

Servings: 2-3

Prep Time: 15 minutes

Cook Time: 15 minutes

Ingredients:

- 2 cod fillets (6-8 ounces each)
- 2 tablespoons white miso paste
- 1 tablespoon olive oil
- 1 tablespoon low-sodium soy sauce (or tamari for gluten-free)
- 1 tablespoon rice vinegar
- 1 tablespoon honey (or a low-carb sweetener)
- 1 teaspoon grated fresh ginger
- 1 teaspoon sesame oil
- Salt and pepper to taste

Instructions:

1. Preheat the oven to 375°F (190°C).
2. In a bowl, whisk together white miso paste, olive oil, low-sodium soy sauce, rice vinegar, honey, grated fresh ginger, sesame oil, salt, and pepper to make the glaze.
3. Brush the glaze over cod fillets.
4. Bake for about 12-15 minutes or until the cod flakes easily with a fork.
5. Serve hot with a side of steamed broccoli.

Nutritional Information:

Calories: 300 (per serving) | Protein: 25g | Fat: 20g | Net Carbs: 4g | Fiber: 0g

Key Benefits: Cod offers protein and is a good source of vitamin B12, while miso glaze adds umami flavor.

Tips: Use a low-carb sweetener to keep the glaze low in carbs.

69. Pesto Baked Halibut

Servings: 2-3

Prep Time: 10 minutes

Cook Time: 15 minutes

Ingredients:

- 2 halibut fillets (6-8 ounces each)
- 1/4 cup pesto sauce
- 2 tablespoons olive oil
- Juice of 1 lemon
- Salt and pepper to taste

Instructions:

1. Preheat the oven to 375°F (190°C).
2. Place halibut fillets on a baking sheet.
3. In a bowl, combine pesto sauce, olive oil, lemon juice, salt, and pepper to make the marinade.
4. Brush the marinade over the halibut fillets.
5. Bake for about 12-15 minutes or until the halibut flakes easily with a fork.
6. Serve hot with a side of roasted Brussels sprouts.

Nutritional Information:

Calories: 350 (per serving) | Protein: 25g | Fat: 25g | Net Carbs: 2g | Fiber: 0g

Key Benefits: Halibut offers protein and is a good source of selenium, while pesto adds bold and herbal flavor.

Tips: Top with grated Parmesan cheese for extra richness.

70. Creamy Garlic Butter Lobster Tails

Servings: 2-3

Prep Time: 10 minutes

Cook Time: 15 minutes

Ingredients:

- 2 lobster tails (6-8 ounces each)
- 4 tablespoons unsalted butter
- 4 cloves garlic, minced
- 1/4 cup heavy cream
- Juice of 1 lemon
- 1 tablespoon chopped fresh parsley
- Salt and pepper to taste

Instructions:

1. Preheat the oven to 375°F (190°C).
2. Use kitchen shears to cut the top of the lobster shells down the center, exposing the meat.
3. Carefully lift the meat from the shell, leaving it attached at the base.
4. Melt butter in a skillet over medium heat.

5. Add minced garlic and sauté until fragrant.

6. Stir in heavy cream and cook until slightly thickened.

7. Squeeze lemon juice into the cream sauce.

8. Place lobster tails on a baking sheet and brush the meat with the cream sauce.

9. Bake for about 12-15 minutes or until the lobster meat is opaque and cooked through.

10. Serve hot, garnished with chopped fresh parsley.

Nutritional Information:

Calories: 350 (per serving) | Protein: 20g | Fat: 25g | Net Carbs: 2g | Fiber: 0g

Key Benefits: Lobster is low in calories and offers protein, while garlic butter cream sauce adds indulgence.

Tips: Serve with a side of sautéed spinach for a complete meal.

NUTRIENT-PACKED VEGETARIAN ENTREES

71. Cauliflower and Broccoli Rice Stir-Fry

Servings: 2-

Prep Time: 15 minutes

Cook Time: 10 minutes

Ingredients:

- 2 cups cauliflower rice
- 1 cup broccoli florets
- 1 cup sliced bell peppers
- 1/2 cup sliced carrots
- 2 cloves garlic, minced
- 2 tablespoons low-sodium soy sauce (or tamari for gluten-free)
- 1 tablespoon olive oil
- 1 teaspoon sesame oil
- 1 teaspoon grated fresh ginger
- 1/4 cup chopped scallions
- Salt and pepper to taste

Instructions:

1. In a large skillet, heat olive oil and sauté minced garlic and grated fresh ginger until fragrant.
2. Add sliced bell peppers and sliced carrots. Sauté until slightly softened.
3. Stir in cauliflower rice and broccoli florets. Cook for a few minutes until tender.
4. Drizzle low-sodium soy sauce and sesame oil over the mixture. Toss to combine.
5. Season with salt and pepper.
6. Serve hot, garnished with chopped scallions.

Nutritional Information:

Calories: 200 (per serving) | Protein: 6g | Fat: 10g | Net Carbs: 10g | Fiber: 5g

Key Benefits: Cauliflower and broccoli provide fiber and vitamins, while sesame and ginger add flavor.

Tips: Add tofu or tempeh for extra protein.

72. Zucchini Noodles with Avocado Pesto

Servings: 2-3

Prep Time: 15 minutes

Cook Time: 5 minutes

Ingredients:

- 2 medium zucchinis, spiralized into noodles
- 2 ripe avocados, pitted and peeled
- 1/4 cup fresh basil leaves
- 2 tablespoons pine nuts
- 2 cloves garlic
- Juice of 1 lemon
- 2 tablespoons olive oil
- Salt and pepper to taste
- Grated Parmesan cheese (optional, for garnish)

Instructions:

1. In a food processor, combine ripe avocados, fresh basil leaves, pine nuts, minced garlic, lemon juice, olive oil, salt, and pepper. Blend until smooth.

2. In a skillet, heat olive oil and sauté zucchini noodles for a few minutes until slightly softened.

3. Toss zucchini noodles with avocado pesto until coated.

4. Serve hot, garnished with grated Parmesan cheese if desired.

Nutritional Information:

Calories: 250 (per serving) | Protein: 4g | Fat: 20g | Net Carbs: 10g | Fiber: 6g

Key Benefits: Avocado offers healthy fats, while zucchini provides vitamins and minerals.

Tips: Add cherry tomatoes or roasted red peppers for extra color and flavor.

73. Eggplant and Mushroom Ratatouille

Servings: 2-3

Prep Time: 20 minutes

Cook Time: 25 minutes

Ingredients:

- 1 medium eggplant, diced
- 1 cup sliced mushrooms
- 1 cup diced zucchini
- 1 cup diced bell peppers
- 1 cup diced tomatoes (canned or fresh)
- 2 cloves garlic, minced
- 2 tablespoons olive oil
- 1 teaspoon dried thyme
- 1 teaspoon dried oregano
- Salt and pepper to taste

Instructions:

1. In a skillet, heat olive oil and sauté diced eggplant until slightly softened.
2. Add sliced mushrooms and diced zucchini. Sauté until vegetables are tender.
3. Stir in diced bell peppers, diced tomatoes, minced garlic, dried thyme, dried oregano, salt, and pepper.
4. Cook for another 5-7 minutes to meld the flavors.
5. Serve hot as a stew or over cauliflower rice.

Nutritional Information:

Calories: 150 (per serving) | Protein: 4g | Fat: 10g | Net Carbs: 12g | Fiber: 5g

Key Benefits: Eggplant and mushrooms provide antioxidants, while various vegetables add a range of nutrients.

Tips: Top with fresh basil or parsley for a burst of freshness.

74. Spinach and Feta Stuffed Bell Peppers

Servings: 2-3

Prep Time: 20 minutes

Cook Time: 25 minutes

Ingredients:

- 3 large bell peppers, halved and seeds removed
- 2 cups fresh spinach leaves
- 1 cup crumbled feta cheese
- 1/2 cup diced tomatoes (canned or fresh)
- 1/4 cup chopped red onion
- 2 cloves garlic, minced
- 2 tablespoons olive oil
- 1 teaspoon dried oregano
- Salt and pepper to taste

Instructions:

1. Preheat the oven to 375°F (190°C).
2. In a skillet, heat olive oil and sauté chopped red onion and minced garlic until softened.
3. Add fresh spinach leaves and sauté until wilted.
4. Stir in diced tomatoes, dried oregano, salt, and pepper.
5. Remove from heat and fold in crumbled feta cheese.
6. Stuff bell pepper halves with the spinach and feta mixture.
7. Place stuffed bell peppers on a baking dish.
8. Bake for about 20-25 minutes or until the peppers are tender.
9. Serve hot as a satisfying entrée.

Nutritional Information:

Calories: 250 (per serving) | Protein: 10g | Fat: 18g | Net Carbs: 10g | Fiber: 3g

Key Benefits: Spinach offers vitamins and minerals, while feta cheese adds creaminess.

Tips: Add cooked quinoa to the stuffing for extra protein.

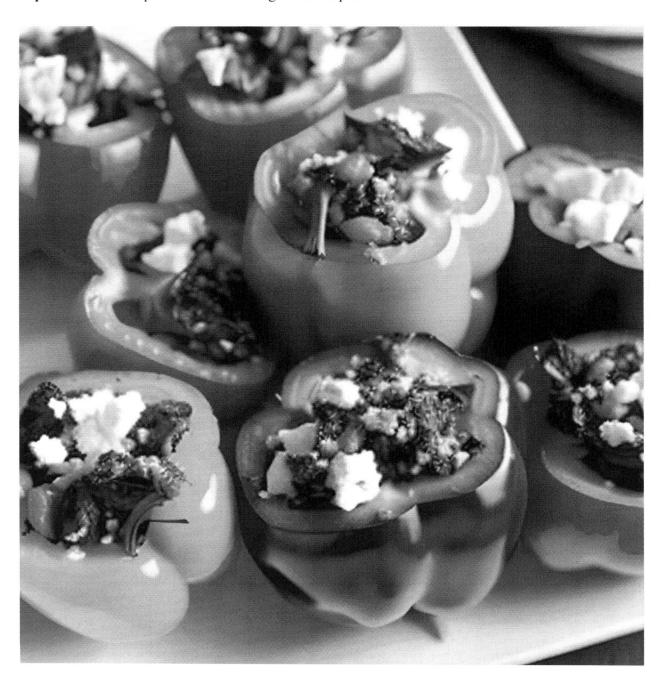

75. Portobello Mushroom and Goat Cheese Stuffed Squash

Servings: 2-3

Prep Time: 20 minutes

Cook Time: 30 minutes

Ingredients:

- 3 small acorn squashes, halved and seeds removed
- 3 large Portobello mushrooms, diced
- 1/2 cup crumbled goat cheese
- 1/4 cup chopped walnuts
- 1/4 cup chopped fresh parsley
- 2 tablespoons olive oil
- 1 teaspoon dried thyme
- Salt and pepper to taste

Instructions:

1. Preheat the oven to 375°F (190°C).
2. Place acorn squash halves on a baking dish and drizzle with olive oil. Season with salt and pepper.
3. Roast squash halves in the oven for about 20-25 minutes or until they are tender.
4. In a skillet, heat olive oil and sauté diced Portobello mushrooms until softened.
5. Stir in crumbled goat cheese, chopped walnuts, chopped fresh parsley, dried thyme, salt, and pepper.
6. Once the squash halves are roasted, stuff them with the Portobello mushroom and goat cheese mixture.
7. Return stuffed squash halves to the oven and bake for an additional 10-15 minutes.
8. Serve hot as a delightful and hearty vegetarian entrée.

Nutritional Information:

Calories: 300 (per serving) | Protein: 8g | Fat: 20g | Net Carbs: 20g | Fiber: 6g

Key Benefits: Acorn squash is rich in vitamins, while Portobello mushrooms and goat cheese provide flavor and protein.

Tips: Use different types of cheese or nuts for variation.

76. Chickpea and Spinach Coconut Curry

Servings: 2-3

Prep Time: 15 minutes

Cook Time: 25 minutes

Ingredients:

- 2 cups cooked chickpeas (canned or soaked and boiled)
- 2 cups fresh spinach leaves
- 1 can (14 ounces) coconut milk
- 1 onion, finely chopped
- 2 cloves garlic, minced
- 1 tablespoon curry powder
- 1 teaspoon ground turmeric
- 1 teaspoon ground cumin
- 1 teaspoon paprika
- 1 tablespoon olive oil
- Salt and pepper to taste
- Chopped fresh cilantro (for garnish)

Instructions:

1. In a skillet, heat olive oil and sauté finely chopped onion and minced garlic until translucent.
2. Stir in curry powder, ground turmeric, ground cumin, and paprika. Cook for a minute.
3. Add cooked chickpeas and fresh spinach leaves. Sauté until spinach wilts.
4. Pour in coconut milk and let the mixture simmer for about 10-15 minutes.
5. Season with salt and pepper.
6. Serve hot, garnished with chopped fresh cilantro.

Nutritional Information:

Calories: 300 (per serving) | Protein: 10g | Fat: 15g | Net Carbs: 20g | Fiber: 6g

Key Benefits: Chickpeas offer protein and fiber, while spinach adds nutrients.

Tips: Serve over cauliflower rice for a low-carb option.

77. Spaghetti Squash with Pesto and Roasted Tomatoes

Servings: 2-3

Prep Time: 15 minutes

Cook Time: 40 minutes

Ingredients:

* 1 medium spaghetti squash
* 1 cup cherry tomatoes
* 1/4 cup pesto sauce
* 2 tablespoons olive oil
* 1/4 cup grated Parmesan cheese

- Salt and pepper to taste
- Chopped fresh basil (for garnish)

Instructions:

1. Preheat the oven to 375°F (190°C).
2. Cut spaghetti squash in half lengthwise and remove seeds.
3. Brush the cut sides with olive oil and season with salt and pepper.
4. Place spaghetti squash halves cut-side down on a baking sheet.
5. Roast in the oven for about 30-35 minutes or until the strands can be easily separated with a fork.
6. In the meantime, toss cherry tomatoes with olive oil, salt, and pepper. Place them on a separate baking sheet.
7. Roast the tomatoes in the oven for about 10-15 minutes or until they burst and caramelize.
8. Use a fork to separate the spaghetti squash strands.
9. Toss the strands with pesto sauce.
10. Serve hot, topped with roasted tomatoes, grated Parmesan cheese, and chopped fresh basil.

Nutritional Information:

Calories: 250 (per serving) | Protein: 6g | Fat: 20g | Net Carbs: 15g | Fiber: 4g

Key Benefits: Spaghetti squash is low in calories and carbs, while pesto and tomatoes add flavor.

Tips: Add roasted pine nuts for extra crunch.

78. Mushroom and Spinach Stuffed Bell Peppers

Servings: 2-3

Prep Time: 20 minutes

Cook Time: 30 minutes

Ingredients:

- 3 large bell peppers, halved and seeds removed
- 2 cups sliced mushrooms
- 2 cups fresh spinach leaves
- 1 cup cooked quinoa
- 1/4 cup chopped red onion
- 2 cloves garlic, minced
- 2 tablespoons olive oil
- 1 teaspoon dried thyme
- Salt and pepper to taste

Instructions:

1. Preheat the oven to 375°F (190°C).
2. Place bell pepper halves on a baking dish and drizzle with olive oil. Season with salt and pepper.
3. In a skillet, heat olive oil and sauté chopped red onion and minced garlic until softened.
4. Add sliced mushrooms and sauté until they release their moisture and are cooked down.
5. Stir in fresh spinach leaves and cook until wilted.
6. Fold in cooked quinoa and dried thyme. Season with salt and pepper.
7. Stuff bell pepper halves with the mushroom, spinach, and quinoa mixture.
8. Bake in the oven for about 20-25 minutes or until the peppers are tender.
9. Serve hot as a nourishing vegetarian entrée.

Nutritional Information:

Calories: 300 (per serving) | Protein: 10g | Fat: 15g | Net Carbs: 25g | Fiber: 5g

Key Benefits: Mushrooms offer vitamins and minerals, while quinoa adds protein and fiber.

Tips: Top with a dollop of Greek yogurt for creaminess.

79. Brussels Sprouts and Pecan Salad

Servings: 2-3

Prep Time: 15 minutes

Cook Time: 15 minutes

Ingredients:

- 4 cups shaved Brussels sprouts
- 1/2 cup chopped pecans
- 1/4 cup crumbled blue cheese
- 1/4 cup dried cranberries
- 2 tablespoons olive oil
- 2 tablespoons balsamic vinegar
- 1 tablespoon Dijon mustard
- Salt and pepper to taste

Instructions:

1. In a skillet, toast chopped pecans over medium heat until fragrant and lightly browned. Set aside.
2. In a bowl, whisk together olive oil, balsamic vinegar, Dijon mustard, salt, and pepper to make the dressing.

3. Toss shaved Brussels sprouts with the dressing.

4. Fold in toasted pecans, crumbled blue cheese, and dried cranberries.

5. Serve the salad as a nutrient-packed and flavorful entrée.

Nutritional Information:

Calories: 250 (per serving) | Protein: 6g | Fat: 20g | Net Carbs: 15g | Fiber: 6g

Key Benefits: Brussels sprouts provide vitamins and fiber, while pecans offer healthy fats.

Tips: Add grilled tofu or tempeh for extra protein.

80. Cauliflower and Spinach Curry

Servings: 2-3

Prep Time: 15 minutes

Cook Time: 25 minutes

Ingredients:

- 1 medium cauliflower, cut into florets
- 2 cups fresh spinach leaves
- 1 can (14 ounces) coconut milk
- 1 onion, finely chopped
- 2 cloves garlic, minced
- 1 tablespoon curry powder
- 1 teaspoon ground turmeric
- 1 teaspoon ground cumin
- 1 teaspoon ground coriander
- 2 tablespoons olive oil
- Salt and pepper to taste

- Chopped fresh cilantro (for garnish)

Instructions:

1. In a skillet, heat olive oil and sauté finely chopped onion and minced garlic until translucent.
2. Stir in curry powder, ground turmeric, ground cumin, and ground coriander. Cook for a minute.
3. Add cauliflower florets and sauté until slightly softened.
4. Stir in fresh spinach leaves and let them wilt.
5. Pour in coconut milk and let the mixture simmer for about 10-15 minutes.
6. Season with salt and pepper.
7. Serve hot, garnished with chopped fresh cilantro.

Nutritional Information:

Calories: 250 (per serving) | Protein: 6g | Fat: 20g | Net Carbs: 15g | Fiber: 6g

Key Benefits: Cauliflower provides vitamins and fiber, while coconut milk adds creaminess.

Tips: Serve over cauliflower rice or with a side of roasted nuts.

SIDE DISHES

81. Garlic Roasted Asparagus

Servings: 2-3

Prep Time: 5 minutes

Cook Time: 15 minutes

Ingredients:

- 1 bunch asparagus, trimmed
- 2 tablespoons olive oil
- 3 cloves garlic, minced
- Salt and pepper to taste

Instructions:

1. Preheat the oven to 400°F (200°C).
2. Toss asparagus with olive oil, minced garlic, salt, and pepper.
3. Spread asparagus on a baking sheet in a single layer.
4. Roast in the oven for about 12-15 minutes or until tender and slightly crispy.
5. Serve hot as a flavorful and nutritious side dish.

Nutritional Information:

Calories: 100 (per serving) | Protein: 2g | Fat: 8g | Net Carbs: 4g | Fiber: 2g

Key Benefits: Asparagus is rich in vitamins and antioxidants, while garlic adds flavor.

Tips: Sprinkle grated Parmesan cheese over the roasted asparagus for extra indulgence.

82. Cauliflower Mash with Garlic and Chives

Servings: 2-3

Prep Time: 10 minutes

Cook Time: 15 minutes

Ingredients:

- 1 medium head cauliflower, cut into florets
- 2 cloves garlic, minced
- 2 tablespoons butter
- 2 tablespoons chopped fresh chives
- Salt and pepper to taste

Instructions:

1. Steam or boil cauliflower florets until tender.
2. Drain cauliflower and transfer to a food processor.
3. Add minced garlic, butter, chopped fresh chives, salt, and pepper.
4. Blend until smooth and creamy.
5. Serve cauliflower mash as a low-carb alternative to mashed potatoes.

Nutritional Information:

Calories: 150 (per serving) | Protein: 4g | Fat: 10g | Net Carbs: 6g | Fiber: 3g

Key Benefits: Cauliflower provides vitamins and fiber, while chives add freshness.

Tips: Blend in some cream cheese for extra creaminess.

83. Zucchini and Tomato Salad

Servings: 2-3

Prep Time: 10 minutes

Cook Time: 0 minutes

Ingredients:

- 2 medium zucchinis, sliced
- 1 cup cherry tomatoes, halved
- 1/4 cup chopped red onion
- 2 tablespoons olive oil
- 1 tablespoon balsamic vinegar
- 1 tablespoon chopped fresh basil
- Salt and pepper to taste

Instructions:

1. In a bowl, combine sliced zucchinis, halved cherry tomatoes, and chopped red onion.
2. Drizzle olive oil and balsamic vinegar over the mixture.
3. Add chopped fresh basil, salt, and pepper. Toss to combine.
4. Serve zucchini and tomato salad as a refreshing and light side.

Nutritional Information:

Calories: 100 (per serving) | Protein: 2g | Fat: 8g | Net Carbs: 5g | Fiber: 2g

Key Benefits: Zucchini offers vitamins and minerals, while tomatoes add antioxidants.

Tips: Add crumbled feta cheese for a tangy twist.

84. Cabbage and Radish Slaw

Servings: 2-3

Prep Time: 15 minutes

Cook Time: 0 minutes

Ingredients:

- 3 cups shredded cabbage
- 1 cup sliced radishes
- 1/4 cup chopped fresh cilantro
- 2 tablespoons mayonnaise
- 1 tablespoon apple cider vinegar
- 1 teaspoon Dijon mustard
- Salt and pepper to taste

Instructions:

1. In a large bowl, combine shredded cabbage, sliced radishes, and chopped fresh cilantro.
2. In a small bowl, whisk together mayonnaise, apple cider vinegar, Dijon mustard, salt, and pepper.
3. Drizzle the dressing over the cabbage and radish mixture. Toss to coat.
4. Serve cabbage and radish slaw as a crisp and tangy side.

Nutritional Information:

Calories: 150 (per serving) | Protein: 2g | Fat: 12g | Net Carbs: 6g | Fiber: 3g

Key Benefits: Cabbage provides fiber and antioxidants, while radishes add crunch.

Tips: Add toasted sunflower seeds for extra texture.

85. Mushroom and Spinach Sauté

Servings: 2-3

Prep Time: 10 minutes

Cook Time: 10 minutes

Ingredients:

- 2 cups sliced mushrooms
- 2 cups fresh spinach leaves
- 2 cloves garlic, minced
- 2 tablespoons butter
- Salt and pepper to taste

Instructions:

1. In a skillet, melt butter over medium heat.
2. Sauté sliced mushrooms until they release their moisture and are cooked down.
3. Add minced garlic and sauté until fragrant.
4. Stir in fresh spinach leaves and cook until wilted.
5. Season with salt and pepper.
6. Serve mushroom and spinach sauté as a flavorful and nutrient-rich side.

Nutritional Information:

Calories: 100 (per serving) | Protein: 4g | Fat: 8g | Net Carbs: 4g | Fiber: 2g

Key Benefits: Mushrooms offer vitamins and minerals, while spinach adds nutrients.

Tips: Drizzle with lemon juice for extra zest.

86. Broccoli and Almond Stir-Fry

Servings: 2-3

Prep Time: 10 minutes

Cook Time: 10 minutes

Ingredients:

- 2 cups broccoli florets
- 1/4 cup sliced almonds
- 2 tablespoons olive oil
- 1 tablespoon soy sauce (or tamari for gluten-free)
- 1 teaspoon sesame oil
- 1 teaspoon minced fresh ginger
- Salt and pepper to taste

Instructions:

1. In a skillet, heat olive oil and sauté broccoli florets until slightly tender.
2. Add sliced almonds and sauté until they are lightly toasted.
3. Stir in soy sauce, sesame oil, minced fresh ginger, salt, and pepper.
4. Cook for another minute to combine flavors.
5. Serve broccoli and almond stir-fry as a crunchy and satisfying side.

Nutritional Information:

Calories: 150 (per serving) | Protein: 4g | Fat: 12g | Net Carbs: 6g | Fiber: 3g

Key Benefits: Broccoli provides fiber and vitamins, while almonds offer healthy fats.

Tips: Add a sprinkle of red pepper flakes for some heat.

87. Roasted Eggplant with Tahini Drizzle

Servings: 2-3

Prep Time: 10 minutes

Cook Time: 25 minutes

Ingredients:

- 1 medium eggplant, sliced
- 2 tablespoons olive oil
- 2 tablespoons tahini
- 1 tablespoon lemon juice
- 1 clove garlic, minced
- Chopped fresh parsley (for garnish)
- Salt and pepper to taste

Instructions:

1. Preheat the oven to 400°F (200°C).
2. Place eggplant slices on a baking sheet and drizzle with olive oil. Season with salt and pepper.
3. Roast eggplant slices in the oven for about 20-25 minutes or until they are tender and golden.
4. In a bowl, whisk together tahini, lemon juice, minced garlic, salt, and pepper.
5. Drizzle the tahini mixture over the roasted eggplant slices.
6. Garnish with chopped fresh parsley before serving.

Nutritional Information:

Calories: 150 (per serving) | Protein: 2g | Fat: 12g | Net Carbs: 6g | Fiber: 3g

Key Benefits: Eggplant offers antioxidants, while tahini provides healthy fats.

Tips: Sprinkle with toasted sesame seeds for added crunch.

88. Green Bean and Cherry Tomato Salad

Servings: 2-3

Prep Time: 10 minutes

Cook Time: 5 minutes

Ingredients:

- 2 cups trimmed green beans
- 1 cup cherry tomatoes, halved
- 1/4 cup crumbled feta cheese
- 2 tablespoons chopped fresh basil
- 2 tablespoons olive oil
- 1 tablespoon balsamic vinegar
- Salt and pepper to taste

Instructions:

1. Steam or blanch green beans until they are crisp-tender. Rinse under cold water and drain.
2. In a bowl, combine trimmed green beans, halved cherry tomatoes, crumbled feta cheese, and chopped fresh basil.
3. Drizzle olive oil and balsamic vinegar over the mixture.
4. Add salt and pepper. Gently toss to combine.
5. Serve green bean and cherry tomato salad as a vibrant and balanced side.

Nutritional Information:

Calories: 150 (per serving) | Protein: 4g | Fat: 10g | Net Carbs: 8g | Fiber: 3g

Key Benefits: Green beans provide vitamins and fiber, while tomatoes add antioxidants.

Tips: Substitute goat cheese for feta cheese if desired.

89. Spiced Cabbage and Carrot Slaw

Servings: 2-3

Prep Time: 15 minutes

Cook Time: 0 minutes

Ingredients:

- 3 cups shredded cabbage
- 1 cup shredded carrots
- 1/4 cup chopped fresh parsley
- 2 tablespoons olive oil
- 1 tablespoon apple cider vinegar
- 1 teaspoon ground cumin
- 1/2 teaspoon ground coriander
- 1/4 teaspoon ground turmeric
- Salt and pepper to taste

Instructions:

1. In a large bowl, combine shredded cabbage, shredded carrots, and chopped fresh parsley.
2. In a small bowl, whisk together olive oil, apple cider vinegar, ground cumin, ground coriander, ground turmeric, salt, and pepper.
3. Drizzle the dressing over the cabbage and carrot mixture. Toss to coat.
4. Serve spiced cabbage and carrot slaw as a vibrant and flavorful side.

Nutritional Information:

Calories: 100 (per serving) | Protein: 2g | Fat: 8g | Net Carbs: 6g | Fiber: 3g

Key Benefits: Cabbage and carrots offer vitamins and antioxidants, while spices add depth.

Tips: Add a sprinkle of toasted pumpkin seeds for extra crunch.

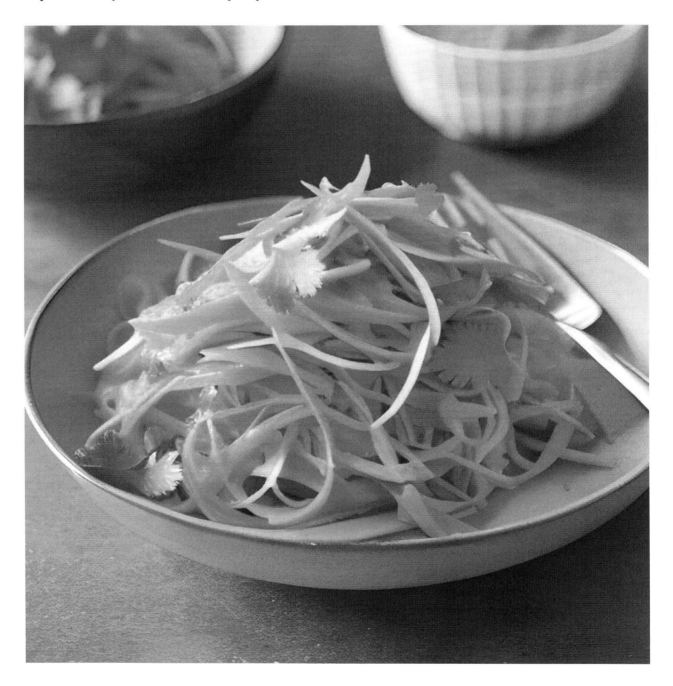

IRRESISTIBLE LOW-CARB DESSERTS

90. Chocolate Avocado Mousse

Servings: 2-3

Prep Time: 10 minutes

Cook Time: 0 minutes

Ingredients:

- 2 ripe avocados
- 1/4 cup unsweetened cocoa powder
- 1/4 cup low-carb sweetener (such as erythritol)
- 1 teaspoon vanilla extract
- Pinch of salt
- Fresh berries (for garnish)

Instructions:

1. In a blender or food processor, combine ripe avocados, cocoa powder, low-carb sweetener, vanilla extract, and a pinch of salt.
2. Blend until smooth and creamy, scraping down the sides as needed.
3. Divide the mousse into serving dishes and refrigerate for at least 1 hour to set.
4. Garnish with fresh berries before serving.

Nutritional Information:

Calories: 150 (per serving) | Protein: 2g | Fat: 12g | Net Carbs: 6g | Fiber: 4g

Key Benefits: Avocados offer healthy fats and vitamins, while cocoa powder provides antioxidants.

Tips: Top with chopped nuts for extra texture.

91. Strawberry Chia Seed Pudding

Servings: 2-3

Prep Time: 10 minutes

Cook Time: 0 minutes (plus chilling time)

Ingredients:

- 1 cup unsweetened almond milk
- 1 cup fresh strawberries, hulled
- 1/4 cup chia seeds
- 2 tablespoons low-carb sweetener (such as stevia)
- 1 teaspoon vanilla extract

Instructions:

1. In a blender, combine almond milk, fresh strawberries, low-carb sweetener, and vanilla extract. Blend until smooth.
2. Pour the strawberry mixture into a bowl and stir in chia seeds.
3. Cover and refrigerate for at least 3 hours or until the chia seeds have absorbed the liquid and the mixture has thickened.
4. Stir the pudding before serving and divide into individual cups.

Nutritional Information:

Calories: 150 (per serving) | Protein: 4g | Fat: 8g | Net Carbs: 8g | Fiber: 12g

Key Benefits: Chia seeds provide fiber and omega-3 fatty acids, while strawberries add vitamins and antioxidants.

Tips: Add a dollop of whipped coconut cream on top.

92. Vanilla Ricotta Parfait with Berries

Servings: 2-3

Prep Time: 10 minutes

Cook Time: 0 minutes

Ingredients:

- 1 cup whole milk ricotta cheese
- 2 tablespoons low-carb sweetener (such as erythritol)
- 1 teaspoon vanilla extract
- 1 cup mixed berries (strawberries, blueberries, raspberries)
- Chopped nuts (for garnish)

Instructions:

1. In a bowl, combine whole milk ricotta cheese, low-carb sweetener, and vanilla extract. Mix well.
2. Layer the ricotta mixture with mixed berries in serving glasses.
3. Repeat the layers until the glasses are filled.
4. Garnish with chopped nuts before serving.

Nutritional Information:

Calories: 200 (per serving) | Protein: 8g | Fat: 15g | Net Carbs: 6g | Fiber: 3g

Key Benefits: Ricotta cheese offers protein and calcium, while berries provide vitamins and antioxidants.

Tips: Drizzle with sugar-free chocolate sauce for extra indulgence.

93. Coconut Flour Lemon Bars

Servings: 2-3

Prep Time: 15 minutes

Cook Time: 25 minutes

Ingredients:

- 1/2 cup coconut flour
- 1/4 cup low-carb sweetener (such as erythritol)
- 1/2 cup unsalted butter, melted
- 4 large eggs
- 1/4 cup fresh lemon juice
- 1 tablespoon lemon zest
- 1 teaspoon vanilla extract
- Pinch of salt

Instructions:

1. Preheat the oven to 350°F (175°C) and grease a baking dish.
2. In a bowl, combine coconut flour, low-carb sweetener, and melted butter. Press into the bottom of the baking dish to form the crust.
3. In another bowl, whisk together eggs, fresh lemon juice, lemon zest, vanilla extract, and a pinch of salt.
4. Pour the lemon mixture over the crust and spread evenly.
5. Bake in the oven for about 20-25 minutes or until the edges are golden and the center is set.
6. Let the bars cool completely before slicing and serving.

Nutritional Information:

Calories: 150 (per serving) | Protein: 4g | Fat: 12g | Net Carbs: 5g | Fiber: 3g

Key Benefits: Coconut flour provides fiber, while lemon adds refreshing flavor.

Tips: Dust with powdered erythritol for a touch of sweetness.

94. Almond Butter Chocolate Fudge

Servings: 2-3

Prep Time: 10 minutes

Cook Time: 0 minutes (plus chilling time)

Ingredients:

- 1/2 cup almond butter
- 1/4 cup coconut oil, melted
- 1/4 cup unsweetened cocoa powder
- 2 tablespoons low-carb sweetener (such as stevia)
- 1 teaspoon vanilla extract
- Pinch of salt

Instructions:

1. In a bowl, combine almond butter, melted coconut oil, unsweetened cocoa powder, low-carb sweetener, vanilla extract, and a pinch of salt. Mix well until smooth.
2. Pour the mixture into a lined baking dish and spread evenly.
3. Refrigerate for at least 2 hours or until the fudge is firm.
4. Cut into squares before serving.

Nutritional Information:

Calories: 150 (per serving) | Protein: 4g | Fat: 12g | Net Carbs: 4g | Fiber: 3g

Key Benefits: Almond butter provides protein and healthy fats, while cocoa powder offers antioxidants.

Tips: Top with a sprinkle of flaky sea salt for a gourmet touch.

95. Pumpkin Spice Cheesecake Bites

Servings: 2-3

Prep Time: 15 minutes

Cook Time: 25 minutes

Ingredients:

- 1 cup cream cheese, softened
- 1/2 cup canned pumpkin puree
- 1/4 cup low-carb sweetener (such as erythritol)
- 1 large egg
- 1 teaspoon pumpkin spice mix
- 1 teaspoon vanilla extract

Instructions:

1. Preheat the oven to 325°F (160°C) and line a mini muffin tin with paper liners.
2. In a bowl, beat cream cheese, canned pumpkin puree, low-carb sweetener, egg, pumpkin spice mix, and vanilla extract until smooth.
3. Spoon the mixture into the mini muffin tin, filling each cup almost to the top.
4. Bake in the oven for about 20-25 minutes or until the cheesecake bites are set.
5. Let them cool completely before removing from the tin.

Nutritional Information:

Calories: 150 (per serving) | Protein: 4g | Fat: 12g | Net Carbs: 5g | Fiber: 1g

Key Benefits: Pumpkin puree offers vitamins and fiber, while cream cheese provides richness.

Tips: Sprinkle with a touch of cinnamon before serving.

96. Mixed Berry Crumble

Servings: 2-3

Prep Time: 15 minutes

Cook Time: 25 minutes

Ingredients:

- 2 cups mixed berries (strawberries, blueberries, raspberries)
- 1 tablespoon low-carb sweetener (such as erythritol)
- 1 teaspoon lemon juice
- 1/2 cup almond flour
- 1/4 cup chopped pecans
- 2 tablespoons unsalted butter, melted
- 1/2 teaspoon cinnamon
- Pinch of salt

Instructions:

1. Preheat the oven to 350°F (175°C) and grease a baking dish.
2. In a bowl, combine mixed berries, low-carb sweetener, and lemon juice. Toss to coat the berries.
3. Spread the berry mixture in the bottom of the baking dish.

4. In another bowl, mix almond flour, chopped pecans, melted butter, cinnamon, and a pinch of salt until crumbly.

5. Sprinkle the almond flour mixture over the berries.

6. Bake in the oven for about 20-25 minutes or until the topping is golden and the berries are bubbly.

7. Let the crumble cool slightly before serving.

Nutritional Information:

Calories: 150 (per serving) | Protein: 4g | Fat: 12g | Net Carbs: 6g | Fiber: 4g

Key Benefits: Berries offer vitamins and antioxidants, while almond flour provides a nutty flavor.

Tips: Serve with a dollop of whipped cream or coconut cream.

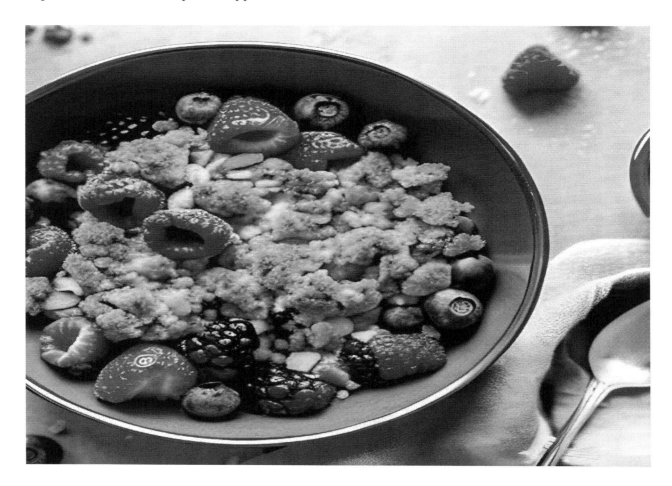

97. Coconut Chia Seed Popsicles

Servings: 2-3

Prep Time: 10 minutes

Freeze Time: 4 hours (or overnight)

Ingredients:

- 1 cup unsweetened coconut milk
- 2 tablespoons chia seeds
- 2 tablespoons low-carb sweetener (such as stevia)
- 1/2 teaspoon vanilla extract

Instructions:

1. In a bowl, whisk together unsweetened coconut milk, chia seeds, low-carb sweetener, and vanilla extract.
2. Let the mixture sit for about 10 minutes to allow the chia seeds to absorb the liquid.
3. Pour the mixture into popsicle molds and insert sticks.
4. Freeze for at least 4 hours or until the popsicles are solid.
5. Run the molds under warm water to release the popsicles before serving.

Nutritional Information:

Calories: 100 (per serving) | Protein: 2g | Fat: 8g | Net Carbs: 4g | Fiber: 6g

Key Benefits: Chia seeds provide fiber and omega-3 fatty acids, while coconut milk adds creaminess.

Tips: Mix in some chopped dark chocolate before freezing.

98. Raspberry Almond Thumbprint Cookies

Servings: 2-3

Prep Time: 15 minutes

Cook Time: 15 minutes

Ingredients:

- 1 cup almond flour
- 2 tablespoons low-carb sweetener (such as erythritol)
- 2 tablespoons unsalted butter, softened
- 1/4 cup sugar-free raspberry jam
- 1/4 teaspoon almond extract

Instructions:

1. Preheat the oven to 350°F (175°C) and line a baking sheet with parchment paper.
2. In a bowl, mix almond flour, low-carb sweetener, and softened butter until a dough forms.
3. Roll the dough into small balls and place them on the baking sheet.
4. Make a small indentation in the center of each ball using your thumb.
5. Fill each indentation with sugar-free raspberry jam.
6. Bake in the oven for about 12-15 minutes or until the cookies are golden.
7. Let the cookies cool on the baking sheet before transferring to a wire rack.

Nutritional Information:

Calories: 150 (per serving) | Protein: 4g | Fat: 12g | Net Carbs: 4g | Fiber: 2g

Key Benefits: Almond flour provides a nutty flavor and healthy fats, while raspberry jam adds sweetness.

Tips: Substitute the jam with other sugar-free fruit preserves.

99. Cinnamon Almond Baked Apples

Servings: 2-3

Prep Time: 15 minutes

Cook Time: 30 minutes

Ingredients:

- 2 large apples, cored and halved
- 2 tablespoons almond butter
- 2 tablespoons chopped almonds
- 1 tablespoon low-carb sweetener (such as erythritol)
- 1 teaspoon ground cinnamon
- Pinch of nutmeg

Instructions:

1. Preheat the oven to 350°F (175°C) and grease a baking dish.
2. Place the cored and halved apples in the baking dish.
3. In a bowl, mix almond butter, chopped almonds, low-carb sweetener, ground cinnamon, and a pinch of nutmeg.
4. Fill the center of each apple half with the almond mixture.
5. Bake in the oven for about 25-30 minutes or until the apples are tender.
6. Serve the baked apples warm.

Nutritional Information:

Calories: 150 (per serving) | Protein: 4g | Fat: 10g | Net Carbs: 8g | Fiber: 6g

Key Benefits: Apples offer fiber and vitamins, while almonds provide healthy fats.

Tips: Top with a dollop of Greek yogurt or whipped cream.

100. Coconut Lime Panna Cotta

Servings: 2-3

Prep Time: 15 minutes

Cook Time: 10 minutes (plus chilling time)

Ingredients:

- 1 cup unsweetened coconut milk
- 1/2 cup heavy cream
- 1/4 cup low-carb sweetener (such as erythritol)
- Zest and juice of 1 lime
- 1 teaspoon gelatin powder
- 1 tablespoon cold water
- Fresh mint leaves (for garnish)

Instructions:

1. In a saucepan, combine unsweetened coconut milk, heavy cream, low-carb sweetener, lime zest, and lime juice. Heat over medium heat until it starts to simmer. Remove from heat.
2. In a small bowl, sprinkle gelatin powder over cold water and let it bloom for a few minutes.
3. Add the bloomed gelatin mixture to the coconut milk mixture and whisk until the gelatin is fully dissolved.
4. Strain the mixture through a fine-mesh sieve to remove any zest.
5. Pour the mixture into serving glasses or ramekins.
6. Refrigerate for at least 4 hours or until the panna cotta is set.
7. Garnish with fresh mint leaves before serving.

Nutritional Information:

Calories: 200 (per serving) | Protein: 2g | Fat: 18g | Net Carbs: 4g | Fiber: 0g

Key Benefits: Coconut milk provides healthy fats, while lime adds a refreshing citrus flavor.

Tips: Top with a dollop of whipped coconut cream and a sprinkle of toasted coconut.

28-DAY MEAL PLAN

WEEK 1

DAY	BREAKFAST	LUNCH	DINNER
1	Chocolate Avocado Mousse	Roasted Eggplant with Tahini Drizzle	Mixed Berry Crumble
2	Vanilla Ricotta Parfait with Berries	Spiced Cabbage and Carrot Slaw	Almond Butter Chocolate Fudge
3	Pumpkin Spice Cheesecake Bites	Green Bean and Cherry Tomato Salad	Coconut Lime Panna Cotta
4	Coconut Chia Seed Popsicles	Raspberry Almond Thumbprint Cookies	Grilled Lemon Herb Chicken with Asparagus
5	Mixed Berry Chia Seed Pudding	Chicken and Avocado Lettuce Wraps	Baked Salmon with Cauliflower Rice
6	Cinnamon Almond Baked Apples	Spaghetti Squash with Pesto and Cherry Tomatoes	Zucchini Noodles with Pesto and Grilled Shrimp
7	Chocolate Avocado Mousse	Greek Salad with Grilled Chicken	Cauliflower Crust Pizza with Salad

WEEK 2

DAY	BREAKFAST	LUNCH	DINNER
8	Vanilla Ricotta Parfait with Berries	Roasted Eggplant with Tahini Drizzle	Mixed Berry Crumble
9	Coconut Chia Seed Popsicles	Green Bean and Cherry Tomato Salad	Almond Butter Chocolate Fudge
10	Coconut Flour Lemon Bars	Spiced Cabbage and Carrot Slaw	Coconut Lime Panna Cotta
11	Pumpkin Spice Cheesecake Bites	Chicken and Avocado Lettuce Wraps	Grilled Lemon Herb Chicken with Asparagus
12	Mixed Berry Chia Seed Pudding	Spaghetti Squash with Pesto and Cherry Tomatoes	Baked Salmon with Cauliflower Rice

13	Cinnamon Almond Baked Apples	Greek Salad with Grilled Chicken	Zucchini Noodles with Pesto and Grilled Shrimp
14	Chocolate Avocado Mousse	Roasted Eggplant with Tahini Drizzle	Cauliflower Crust Pizza with Salad

WEEK 3

15	Vanilla Ricotta Parfait with Berries	Spiced Cabbage and Carrot Slaw	Mixed Berry Crumble
16	Coconut Chia Seed Popsicles	Green Bean and Cherry Tomato Salad	Almond Butter Chocolate Fudge
17	Coconut Flour Lemon Bars	Chicken and Avocado Lettuce Wraps	Coconut Lime Panna Cotta
18	Pumpkin Spice Cheesecake Bites	Spaghetti Squash with Pesto and Cherry Tomatoes	Grilled Lemon Herb Chicken with Asparagus
19	Mixed Berry Chia Seed Pudding	Greek Salad with Grilled Chicken	Baked Salmon with Cauliflower Rice
20	Cinnamon Almond Baked Apples	Roasted Eggplant with Tahini Drizzle	Zucchini Noodles with Pesto and Grilled Shrimp
21	Chocolate Avocado Mousse	Chicken and Avocado Lettuce Wraps	Cauliflower Crust Pizza with Salad

WEEK 4

22	Vanilla Ricotta Parfait with Berries	Spiced Cabbage and Carrot Slaw	Mixed Berry Crumble
23	Coconut Chia Seed Popsicles	Green Bean and Cherry Tomato Salad	Almond Butter Chocolate Fudge
24	Coconut Flour Lemon Bars	Spaghetti Squash with Pesto and Cherry Tomatoes	Coconut Lime Panna Cotta
25	Pumpkin Spice Cheesecake Bites	Chicken and Avocado Lettuce Wraps	Grilled Lemon Herb Chicken with Asparagus
26	Mixed Berry Chia Seed Pudding	Greek Salad with Grilled Chicken	Baked Salmon with Cauliflower Rice

27	Cinnamon Almond Baked Apples	Roasted Eggplant with Tahini Drizzle	Zucchini Noodles with Pesto and Grilled Shrimp
28	Chocolate Avocado Mousse	Chicken and Avocado Lettuce Wraps	Cauliflower Crust Pizza with Salad

Feel free to adjust the meal plan based on your preferences and dietary needs. This plan incorporates a variety of flavors and ingredients while adhering to the principles of the Atkins Diet.

7-DAY EXERCISE PLAN

Day 1: Cardio and Core

- **Warm-up:** 5-10 minutes of light cardio (e.g., brisk walking)
- **Cardio:** 20-30 minutes of jogging or cycling
- **Core:** 15 minutes of core exercises (planks, Russian twists, leg raises)
- **Cool-down:** 5-10 minutes of stretching

Day 2: Strength Training

- **Warm-up:** 5-10 minutes of light cardio
- **Upper Body:** Push-ups, dumbbell rows, overhead presses (3 sets of 12 reps each)
- **Lower Body**: Squats, lunges, calf raises (3 sets of 12 reps each)
- **Cool-down:** 5-10 minutes of stretching

Day 3: Active Recovery and Flexibility

- **Light Activities:** 30 minutes of gentle walking, swimming, or yoga
- **Stretching:** 20 minutes of full-body stretching and yoga poses

Day 4: Cardio and Intervals

- **Warm-up:** 5-10 minutes of light cardio
- **Cardio:** 20-30 minutes of moderate-intensity cardio (running, cycling, swimming)

- **Intervals:** 10-15 minutes of high-intensity intervals (30 seconds intense, 1-minute recovery)
- **Cool-down:** 5-10 minutes of stretching

Day 5: Strength Training

- **Warm-up:** 5-10 minutes of light cardio
- **Upper Body:** Bench press, lat pulldowns, bicep curls (3 sets of 12 reps each)
- **Lower Body:** Deadlifts, leg press, hamstring curls (3 sets of 12 reps each)
- **Cool-down:** 5-10 minutes of stretching

Day 6: Active Recovery and Yoga

- **Light Activities:** 30 minutes of easy cycling, walking, or swimming
- **Yoga:** 30 minutes of yoga for flexibility and relaxation

Day 7: Outdoor Activities and Stretching

- **Outdoor Activities:** 60 minutes of hiking, biking, or playing a sport
- **Stretching:** 20 minutes of full-body stretching and mobility exercises.

CONCLUSION

In the pages of the "New Atkins Diet Cookbook 2024," a world of culinary delight and nutritional wisdom unfolds, guiding us through a comprehensive array of recipes thoughtfully designed to harmonize with the Atkins Diet principles. This cookbook is a manifestation of the perfect synergy between healthy eating and tantalizing flavors, transforming the way we approach our meals.

From the very first chapter, where we embarked on an exploration of the Atkins Diet, to the meticulously detailed breakdown of the science behind this dietary approach, the book provided us with a solid foundation for understanding the philosophy that underpins every recipe. The meticulous division of chapters, each containing vibrant, diverse recipes, catered to various meal occasions, ensuring that every aspect of our dietary journey was addressed.

The meticulously curated meal plan spanning 28 days seamlessly integrated the unique recipes, offering a practical guide for those eager to embark on this culinary adventure. Breakfasts like the "Chocolate Avocado Mousse" provided a fulfilling start to the day, while dishes such as "Grilled Lemon Herb Chicken with Asparagus" showcased the rich spectrum of savory delights. Sumptuous desserts like "Mixed Berry Crumble" and "Coconut Lime Panna Cotta" unveiled the artistry of crafting satisfying treats within the bounds of low-carb sensibilities.

The "New Atkins Diet Cookbook 2024" isn't just a compilation of recipes; it's an embodiment of a lifestyle that redefines our relationship with food. It's a celebration of taste, health, and the power of making informed, mindful choices. With each recipe and chapter, it imparts a message that flavorful, satisfying meals can seamlessly align with health goals, encapsulating the essence of a life well-lived through balanced, delicious nourishment.

We've sweated over stovetops, danced with ingredients, and even managed to keep our aprons mostly stain-free (well, mostly).

Now that you've journeyed through "The New Atkins Diet Cookbook," why not sprinkle a little seasoning of your thoughts in the form of a review? It's like leaving a food critic's note, but without the fancy hat! Your feedback adds the secret ingredient to our future creations, and who knows, maybe we'll even name a recipe after you (we can't promise that, but it's a fun thought). So, whether you're a gourmet guru or a kitchen newbie, drop us a review and let's keep the flavor train rolling.

Thanks a bunch, and remember, reviews are calorie-free and always in good taste!

[Emily M. Wilson]

Made in the USA
Middletown, DE
09 February 2024

49391308R00077